The Nature of Suffering and the Goals of Nursing

The Nature of Suffering
and the Goals of Nursing

Betty R. Ferrell
Nessa Coyle

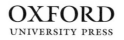

OXFORD
UNIVERSITY PRESS

2008

OXFORD

UNIVERSITY PRESS

Oxford University Press, Inc., publishes works that further
Oxford University's objective of excellence
in research, scholarship, and education.

Oxford   New York
Auckland   Cape Town   Dar es Salaam   Hong Kong   Karachi
Kuala Lumpur   Madrid   Melbourne   Mexico City   Nairobi
New Delhi   Shanghai   Taipei   Toronto

With offices in
Argentina   Austria   Brazil   Chile   Czech Republic   France   Greece
Guatemala   Hungary   Italy   Japan   Poland   Portugal   Singapore
South Korea   Switzerland   Thailand   Turkey   Ukraine   Vietnam

Copyright © 2008 by Oxford University Press, Inc.

Published by Oxford University Press, Inc.
198 Madison Avenue, New York, New York 10016

www.oup.com

Library of Congress Cataloging-in-Publication Data
Ferrell, Betty,
The nature of suffering and the goals of nursing / Betty R. Ferrell, Nessa Coyle
    p.   ;   cm.
ISBN: 978-0-19-533312-1 (pbk.)
1. Nursing—Philosophy.   2. Suffering.
3. Nurse and patient.   I. Ferrell, Betty.   II. Title.
[DNLM: 1. Nursing Care.   2. Terminal Care.   3. Nurses—psychology.
4. Pain—nursing.   5. Palliative Care. WY 152 C881n 2008]
RT84.5.C69 2008
610.7301—dc22   2007034156

9 8 7 6 5 4 3 2 1

Printed in the United States of America
on acid-free paper

This book is dedicated to Dr. Kathleen Foley, a friend, colleague and compassionate physician who has devoted her life to the care of the dying and their families. Dr. Foley has long been a forceful advocate for nurses and opened many doors in an era when such doors were closed. She is an extraordinary woman, not only for her intellect and advocacy for the dying and the disadvantaged, but especially because of her simple humanity has not gotten lost along the way
    —Thank you, Kathy.

PREFACE

In a recent visit overseas, a nurse recounted a story to one of the authors (Nessa Coyle) of a dying child on a respirator who was neither sedated nor given pain medication because of the fear that the child's death might be hastened. This possibility went against all religious beliefs of the community, although the individual child's suffering caused anguish and questioning among the nursing and medical staff.

The nurse caring for the child described the child's eyes as pleading to her to allow death to come, but that she could do nothing to alleviate his suffering. A colleague advised her to avoid the child's eyes and in that way she would be able to continue to care for him.

Although this example may appear extreme, it is not unusual. Staying by the side of chronically ill and dying individuals, adults or children, who may be experiencing unremitting pain, difficulty in breathing, confusion, loss of meaning, despair, and/or overwhelming grief is what nurses do. Sometimes they have the tools to relieve or ameliorate the suffering, sometimes not. But they are always a presence.

The essence of nursing care continually exposes nurses to suffering. Although they bear witness to the suffering of others, their own suffering is less frequently exposed. This slim volume attempts to give voice to the suffering nurses witness in patients, families, colleagues, and themselves. By making this suffering visible, we honor it and may learn from it.

ACKNOWLEDGMENTS

The authors acknowledge the pioneering work on suffering by Eric Cassell and the gracious sharing of his work as a foundation for our work. We also acknowledge the review and contributions of several colleagues in the preparation of this book. We are grateful for the wisdom of Tami Borneman, Hob Osterlund, Hollye Harrington Jacobs, Mary Jo Prince-Paul, Catherine Wagar, and Ken Zuroski. We also greatly appreciate all of the patients and families whose stories are reflected here. We hope this book is a guide for nurses as they do the daily work of our profession—the relief of suffering.

Betty Ferrell acknowledges the incredible wisdom and guidance of her thesis committee at Claremont Graduate University, Dr. Ellen Marshall and Dr. Kathleen Greider.

We also acknowledge the editorial assistance of Chan Thai and Andrea Hayward, who worked diligently through every phase of this book to make it a reality.

CONTENTS

The Nature of Suffering and
the Goals of Nursing

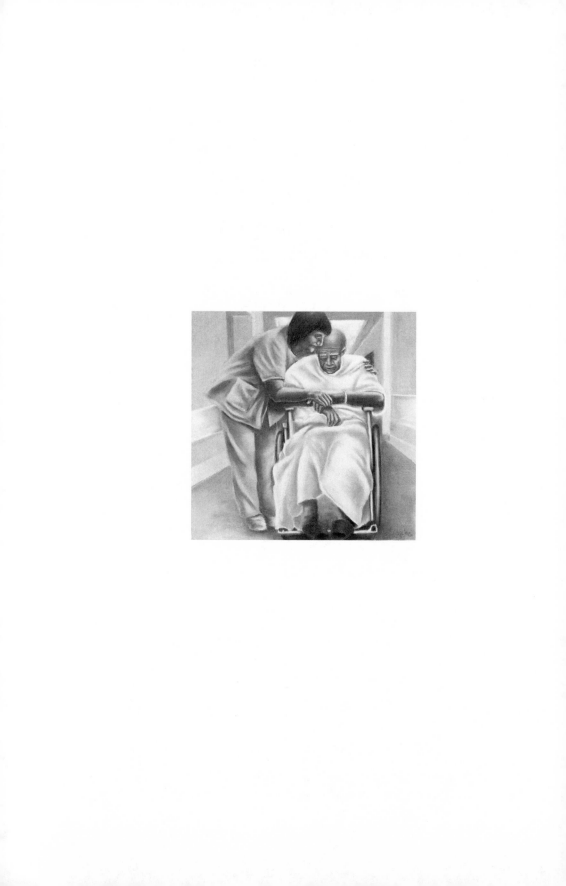

CHAPTER 1 ✺

Suffering and the Practice
of Nursing

✺

In a medical–surgical unit in a small Midwestern hospital, a patient's suffering is reduced by the night-shift nurse. The elderly woman has lung cancer. She was admitted 2 days prior with a bowel obstruction, likely the cumulative result of immobility, inadequate food and fluid intake, medication side effects, and progressive disease. Her uncontrollable nausea, vomiting, and pain over the past few days at home are now relieved by a nasogastric (NG) tube, intravenous (IV) fluids, and careful titration of analgesics. Having finally slept a few hours, the woman awakens in the middle of the night. Given the myriad of tubes and wires attached to her body, she remains motionless, afraid to move. Still, her wakefulness stirs her exhausted daughter wedged into a reclining chair at her bedside.

Mother and daughter exchange mutual queries: "Are you okay?" "Why don't you go home?" the mother suggests. "This chair is fine," the daughter lies. The woman's husband went home after a few hours at the hospital. After 55 years of marriage, the angst of seeing his wife so miserably ill and the strangeness of the hospital world were enough to propel him home, despite the silence and loneliness of an empty house. Mother and daughter reaffirm to each other that he's home asleep, but both know he is probably wide awake, sitting in his easy chair in the living room, sipping stale coffee, reading his Bible, and counting on God to come through. After all, God has come through many times before. He has faith. God will come through again.

The night nurse enters the room, careful not to turn on the bright lights even though she sees that both mother and daughter are awake. She performs the routine checks—NG tube functioning, IV dripping, urinary catheter draining. The same nurse was on duty when the woman was admitted the night before. Comparing her patient's distress then and her current relatively peaceful state, and given the goals of care, she decides to skip the routine vital signs. Instead, she asks the woman how she's doing. The woman politely answers, "Fine." She adds that she didn't really know how bad she had felt until she started to feel better.

The nurse resists the urge to hurry out the door to the next patient and continue her long list of tasks. It is hard to stand still. She sees the woman's cachectic body, she hears the flow of oxygen and the pulsing suction of the NG tube, and she feels the clammy coolness of the woman's arm as she gently touches it. The nurse knows well the signs of approaching death. Too well. Death is a frequent visitor here in the hospital.

Assured of her patient's comfort, the nurse speaks to the daughter, "You must be relieved your mother is not in pain now." The nurse says how wonderful it is that the daughter has been able to be here and acknowledges the daughter's exhaustion. As the daughter's eyes fill with tears, she finds herself grateful that the room is dark. In just 2 days, she will need to leave to pack her own daughter for college. On the airplane, she will reverse roles, become the mother, and somehow navigate this other—and almost as difficult—rite of passage. After the move to college is completed, her husband will drop her off at the closest airport so she can return to her mother. She's been praying a lot. She asks God whose idea this is that she may lose her mother and daughter in the same week. Her faith is usually strong, but not this week. She's found her limit.

The nurse senses the quiet tears of the daughter, hidden from her mother's eyes as she lies next to her, staring at the dark ceiling. She asks the daughter if she would like some coffee. It is the mother who answers, "We are tea sippers." She describes how the two of them had "tea parties" all their lives. From the time the daughter was a little girl with a floral porcelain tea set to the current heartier mugs shared over monumental life decisions, the two have sipped tea. The pale and weak patient perks up and proclaims, "You know, we could have a tea party now!"

The nurse hesitates. The woman is "NPO," indicating she can't have oral fluids due to the bowel obstruction. But given that the primary goal for her patient is comfort, and given the enormous pleasure this ritual would give them, the nurse decides to let her have a few sips of tea. The NG suction will keep the sips from becoming instant, violent nausea. In silence all three women realize with profound grief that this tea party may well be the last. The nurse excuses herself and goes to go to her locker to get a "special stash" tea bag. No industrial hospital tea bag will do, not for this occasion.

She returns in a moment. A full cup for the daughter, another smaller cup and a straw for the patient. There is a deliberate pause, then an intimate connection as the nurse's hand touches the daughter's hand and lingers as she offers the tea. She leaves only when she is certain her patient is comfortable, careful to leave the lights off and to close the door quietly. The mother and daughter sip tea. In the stillness of the room, with only the intermittent sound of the suction machine, they are recipients of the sacred care of a nurse.

This case illustrates the nature of suffering and the goals of nursing. On one level, the story is a very simple narrative of a common situation. On another level, it is a rich and deep portrayal of the work of nursing delivered at one of the most poignant moments in the lives of a mother and her daughter. This deep and profound experience of suffering is the focus of this book.

CASSELL'S FOUNDATIONAL WORK ON THE NATURE OF SUFFERING

In 1982, Eric Cassell, M.D., published a seminal paper on suffering. The insightful voice of this paper, and its appearance in the *New England Journal of Medicine*, opened the door to what has become an ongoing professional conversation about suffering in health-care settings (Cassell, 1982). Cassell's original article was later expanded to a book, and his initial paper has been cited internationally by professionals from many disciplines, thus challenging systems to respond not only to physical injury and disease but also to human suffering (Cassell, 1991, 1999).

The essence of Cassell's description is that suffering is "experienced by persons, not merely by bodies, and has its source in challenges that threaten the intactness of the person as a complex social and psychologic entity" (Cassell, 1982). Cassell also stated that suffering may include pain but is not limited to it, and the relief of suffering is an *obligation* of medicine. Cassell's classic paper should be required reading for all health-care professionals. His comparisons of pain versus suffering and his exploration of the concept of *meaning* echo the historic themes of medicine and nursing. Although both disciplines have a professional mandate to relieve suffering, the current status of health care often fails to uphold this basic tenet. Nursing and medicine have become highly technical and often very depersonalized.

Cassell's analysis of the meaning of illness is particularly relevant to nursing. He described *personal meaning* as a fundamental dimension of personhood and stated that the act of recognizing personal meaning is critical to understanding human illness and suffering. He also faulted modern medicine for ignoring the transcendent dimension—the spirit of human life.

Cassell's criticisms of the medical profession and his challenge to physicians to respond to human suffering apply equally to nursing. Nurses have evolved from the highly personalized care modeled by founder Florence Nightingale (who organized a unit of 38 women in 1854 for service in the Crimean War) to a modern-day bedside characterized by high-tech equipment, alarms, and digital data. In modern health care, financial implications commonly override considerations of individual needs. This highly structured, technical, and reimbursement-driven environment couldn't be further from Nightingale's emphasis on personal touch, fresh air, and silence.

Nurses and physicians are, at their core, compassionate and dedicated professionals who want to do good. But "doing good" has become difficult and more complex. When Cassell wrote his textbook *The Nature of Suffering and the Goals of Medicine* (1991), he censured modern medicine for not only failing to relieve suffering but for often actually *intensifying* suffering. What happened? Why have advances in medicine and nursing moved us further from, not closer to, recognizing and treating suffering? When nurses ask such fundamental questions as "What is the nature of suffering?" and "What are the goals of nursing?" we also must consider the paradox of our own professional advances contrasted with human disconnection and unrelieved suffering—even unrecognized or intensified human suffering.

NURSING EDUCATION AND SUFFERING

A few years ago, a review of 50 leading textbooks in nursing was conducted as preliminary research on end-of-life care and nursing education. Parallel work was being performed in medicine. Review of 45,000 pages of nursing texts revealed that only 2% of the content was devoted to any topic related to end-of-life care (Ferrell, Virani, and Grant, 1999). Even the pain-management content, which one might assume to be a fundamental concern of nursing, was largely absent or often abysmally incorrect.

As a means of follow-up to the initial review of the textbooks, a conference was organized and held in San Francisco with medical and nursing authors, editors, and publishers to award those who had improved end-of-life care content in texts. I (Betty Ferrell) arrived early for the meeting and decided to take a stroll downtown. On my walk I came upon an antique bookshop that had a nursing text from the early 1900s. Intrigued and amused, I looked up "pain" and "end-of-life care" in the index. What I found surprised me. There was correct information and significant detail. The book encouraged nurses to accept pain relief as a mandate. To be a good nurse was to be sure your patient was not in pain. I couldn't help but ask myself where we deviated from this mandate. I couldn't help but think that in our "progress" over the last century we have abandoned some of our basic professional obligations. At the textbook publishers' meeting a few hours later, I read from this text to illustrate that our progress in nursing was perhaps, in some ways, not progress at all.

Another vital concern is the reality that nurses often actually *inflict* pain through various procedures, such as inserting IV lines, wound debridement, tracheostomy suctioning, and a myriad of other clinical functions. A doctoral nursing dissertation by Irena Madjar, "Giving Comfort and Inflicting Pain" (1998), explored the experiences of nurses as they faced the dichotomy of both relieving pain and, at times, being an agent of pain or suffering. This dissonance between causing and relieving pain is also felt in a nurse's moral disquiet when she administers a dose of morphine to an imminently dying patient out of a desire to relieve pain but with a concern that the medication itself may hasten death. Every day, the nurses in neonatal intensive care units (ICU) weigh the costs and benefits of using technical expertise that allows them to perform painful procedures on the smallest and most vulnerable of infants. Every day, nurses in emergency departments, trauma centers, burn centers, and other intensive care settings work desperately to save lives and are often required to inflict pain and discomfort. Inflicting this pain may be considered a necessary act—especially when attempts to save life are successful—but may become a memory of inflicting torture if efforts to rescue fail and patients die.

The essence of this question can be illustrated through our experiences in national efforts to improve nursing education and end-of-life care. In developing the End of Life Nursing Education Consortium (ELNEC), investigators at the City of Hope National Medical Center and the American Association of Colleges of Nursing began by conducting descriptive research to establish current nursing practice in end-of-life care. This descriptive work included surveys of practicing nurses, faculty, and deans of schools of nursing (Ferrell, Grant, and Virani, 1999; Ferrell, Virani, and Grant, 1999; Ferrell, Virani, Grant, Coyne, and Uman, 2000). The foundational work of the ELNEC project included the previously described review of leading nursing textbooks and national evaluation of nursing school curricula. The ELNEC research was important to create a baseline of the status of nursing education before implementing improvements. Recognizing that our initial findings indicated significant need for improvement, we were especially interested in the response from some nursing skeptics who asked "Don't nurses already know this?" or who suggested that although medicine might need support in end-of-life care, "Surely *nurses* are already doing good care, aren't they?"

The results of these descriptive studies were powerful and revealing. Nursing schools had little focus on end-of-life care overall and even more limited focus on the most basic topics, such as pain. Students have routinely graduated and entered practice never having cared for a dying patient, only to assume a job as a new graduate on an oncology unit or other clinical setting where death is common. Nurses in clinical practice have described inadequacy in managing pain, inability to communicate with dying patients and their families, as well as their own moral distress resulting from participation in what they considered futile care.

This incongruity between nursing education and nursing practice exacts a toll on nurses, which undoubtedly contributes to professional stress, personal distress, and the consideration of alternative professions. The following case example illustrates this incongruity:

A senior nursing student becomes interested in critical care as a career option and focuses her clinical and classroom time on mastering the knowledge and skills needed to work in this area. She feels jubilant in getting a coveted position as a new nurse in a medical ICU reserved for only a few new graduates. She has a 4-month internship and continues to work on mastering the necessary skills for her job: doing a physical exam, knowing complex pharmacology, interpreting lab data, and meticulously assessing and responding to rapid change in the multisystem disease course of her patients.

But then the disconnect begins. The nurse is now well-prepared to assess, monitor, respond, and communicate with colleagues about the physiologic events in critically ill patients. But she is ill-prepared to deal with the daily work of responding to pain, anxiety, spiritual crisis, hopelessness, and fear. Most importantly, the nurse has not yet learned

how to deal with a common statistic in intensive care settings: 20%–
30% of her patients will die in this hospitalization. She will not know
what to do when the intubated, terrified man mouths the words, "Am I
dying?" or the timid grandmother reaches for her hand and says,
"Please, take care of my grandson. I pray you will save him. He is so
young."

Nursing education and the support systems to sustain nurses in practice must surround technical proficiency with human compassion. Nursing care is always performed in relationship with two people: one a caring nurse and another a human in need of support.

DEFINING SUFFERING

Nurses have defined suffering in various ways, capturing the essence of patients' experiences as they face serious illness and death. Table 1.1 summarizes definitions of suffering provided by nurses. These definitions capture not only the experiences of patients but also the intense emotions of nurses as they stand witness to such suffering. In many of these examples, it is difficult to determine whether the nurses are describing their own suffering or that which they observe in others.

In 1971, Travelbee explored both suffering as a unique human experience and the response of nurses to those who suffer (Travelbee, 1971). Laurel Copp, a pioneer in nursing perspectives on the topic of suffering, defined suffering as "a state of anguish in one who bears pain, injury, or loss" (Copp, 1974, 1990a, 1990b). Copp and Travelbee were among the first nursing scholars to recognize opportunities for nurses to respond to suffering through their intimate relationships with patients.

There are specific skills nurses can acquire in their response to suffering, such as therapeutic communication and active listening, to discover the actual source of suffering. The essential task of nursing, echoed throughout this text, is mastering the art of presence. Simply being *present* in the face of suffering is a basic, yet profoundly complex, act (Battenfield, 1984; Coyle, 1996, 2004).

The historical perspective of illness as only a physical event ignores the reality that most chronic and life-threatening diseases become whole-person experiences that inevitably include suffering. An example of the reductionist approach to illness can be seen in examining the symptom of fatigue. In oncology, fatigue had often been viewed as simply a side effect of treatment, a transient symptom easily relieved or at least improved by sleep,

Table 1.1. Definitions of Suffering from Nurses

Multidimensional Distress

Suffering—an inner distress. It's the deep down inner-most self, placed at the bottom of the barrel, and when crisis hits home, those bottom-of-the-barrel thoughts filter to the top. It is real, it can be painful, it can be the realization of things you have done or have NOT done and now, with wisdom, you realize they were wrong or hurt someone you love—it can stir up so much.

Grief/Loss

It is quietly knowing loss—loss of possessions, loss of abilities, loss of those you love, and possibly, loss of self.

To suffer is to experience loss: of comfort, of familiarity, a body part, a sense of safety, a sense of what is known, of what defines home, of personal story, and identity.

Multidimensional Pain

Suffering means to me to be in unbearable emotional or physical pain—to be in a situation that you feel trapped in, to be without hope, would be the deepest sense of suffering.

Multidimensional Discomfort

It means there exists within a person a sense of deep intense discomfort, whether physical or emotional. It's accompanied by some degree of helplessness and hopelessness. It is to hurt.

Loss of Control/Helplessness

We suffer when we are faced with elements or conditions in our environment that we feel powerless to change.

Not getting relief from pain—deep distress from not being heard. Being coerced to do treatment when the patient does not want to. Being told, "You will die if you don't do this."

Hopelessness

Having no hope, even in death . . . Not having any control over your situation . . .

Inability to Cope

Not being able to say, "I'm dying and that's okay" . . . desperately needing those you love to talk about it and to touch you and hold you.

To suffer deeply is to resist loss, deny its reality, to need to be in charge of that which cannot be controlled, to lose humor, and to believe oneself alone and abandoned.

A Personal Experience

Suffering is multidimensional and the expert in the true meaning of suffering is the person who is suffering.

Suffering is a word that can be defined by each individual with his or her own experience.

(continued)

Table 1.1. (*continued*)

Anxiety/Worry/Restlessness/Lack of Peace

In a dying patient it probably encompasses spiritual, emotional, financial, pain, and symptom issues. Suffering is not feeling at peace with oneself.

Isolation/Loneliness/Depression

. . . Suffering is being alone in thoughts and feelings, wanting desperately to share them but fearing to admit what is felt or unknown; wanting to protect others, wanting to protect self. Suffering is often more than can be put into words yet screaming to be disclosed.

and not as serious as pain or other urgent syndromes. Complaints of fatigue were often ignored, or are met with a response such as, "Of course you are tired," or by a dismissal that the symptom will "go away" or "it is expected." An even more distressing response sometimes described by patients is to hear a nurse or physician say, "You think *you're* tired? I'm exhausted!" implying that the health-care provider's exhaustion from a busy clinic schedule could compare to the profound fatigue associated with the life-threatening disease of cancer and its treatment.

To gain a deeper understanding of the phenomenon of fatigue, research conducted at the City of Hope National Medical Center analyzed descriptions of patients' fatigue according to a quality-of-life (QOL) model that included physical, psychological, social, and spiritual domains (Ferrell, Grant, Dean, Funk, and Ly, 1996). This analysis revealed meanings of the physical problem of fatigue and illustrated the intense and profound impact of this "side effect" on patient suffering. Table 1.2 includes descriptions of fatigue from this study. The words illustrate the patients' distress and remind us that a physical problem can become an all-consuming experience demanding urgent care that addresses all dimensions of QOL. These descriptions of fatigue include a forced change in priorities, a crippling of previous spiritual or religious beliefs, hopelessness, challenges in coping, depression, and anxiety.

The phenomenon of fatigue impacting QOL is depicted in Figure 1.1. A multidimensional analysis of fatigue may also be applied to many other symptoms or side effects of diseases or treatments. For example, nausea associated with chronic gastrointestinal disease often quickly moves from being an inconvenient or irritating physical concern to an all-consuming experience. Weight loss accompanying chronic nausea or anorexia becomes a symptom that causes devastating body image changes and a cascade of other symptoms.

The model (Figure 1.1) depicts how a treatment such as cancer chemotherapy causes physiologic effects, which in turn cause the symptom

Table 1.2. Patient Descriptions of Fatigue Illustrating Suffering

Changes in Spirituality

I expect so much of myself but deep down I know I can only give of myself so very little. The spiritual side of life is present in me now much more so than before I knew I had a devastating disease.

My learning in a nutshell, which surprised me, has been that while I had a very difficult time removing myself from my world as I knew it, leading a greatly simplified life with only work and singing in a choir as I had energy, reentering the world after 9-10 months of quiet reflection was just as difficult. I realized how my time of reflection had indeed changed me. It has left me both with a sense of urgency to go forward and live each day fully as well as a renewed sense of how important time for reflection is to my well-being. I experienced patience and reflected on the scripture when Jesus says, "I give you my peace, not as the world knows it."

Changed Priorities/Sense of Time

It has been a deterrent at times to living fully, especially during treatment. Fatigue wastes time and time seems precious.

Hopelessness

For me I feel that I have fought enough, given enough, lost enough. I'm tired of having to struggle just to survive while watching others take it for granted. Sometimes it's easier to look upon my cancer as a curse. When I do find myself feeling low I try to look upon my battles as a gift of sorts. Because I have had to fight so hard to live, I have been blessed with an appreciation of life that only us survivors can achieve.

Coping/Acceptance

I used to rule my body—now my body rules me. It tells me when to lie down and relax and there's no more "pushing my body."

Depression and Anxiety

. . . I was reduced to being dependent, incapable. I felt incapable. Although I had to keep up all my responsibilities, you know the responsibilities don't change. I'm sick and tired and I had to do those things. So, it was just like getting through. And that mentality gets old. You get depressed.

Adapted with permission from Ferrell, B.R., M. Grant, G. E. Dean, B. Funk, and J. Ly. 1996. "Bone Tired": The Experience of Fatigue and Its Impact on Quality of Life. *Oncology Nursing Forum*, 23:1539–1547.

(patient experience) of fatigue. The result of the patient experience is impact on all dimensions of QOL, including physical, psychological, social, and spiritual well-being. The cumulative impact of these concerns increases the patient's suffering. More importantly, the suffering that is experienced counterinfluences each dimension of QOL.

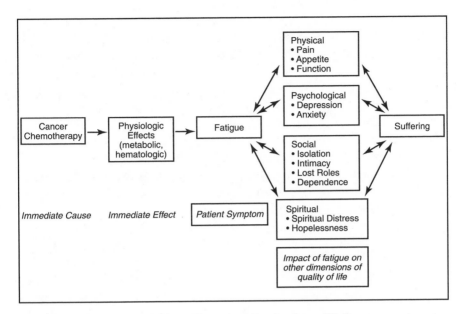

Figure 1.1. The Process of Fatigue Impacting Quality of Life

Another common oncology symptom is alopecia, or hair loss. The loss of one's hair, easily explained in physiologic terms as a result of chemotherapeutic agents, is commonly an early manifestation of suffering, even if the patient's prognosis for survival is good. It is also an example of a symptom that is not physically painful but may be spiritually devastating. The loss of one's hair is often described as a profound moment of recognition that the cancer is real, that death is possible, and that the person has at least momentarily lost control. This is a suffering that begins not at the transition from chronic to terminal illness (when suffering is more commonly expected), but rather at the transition from health to initial diagnosis of illness (Ferrell and Sun, 2006).

The experience of suffering from symptoms of disease or treatment is by no means limited to oncology. Figure 1.1 could equally be applied to dyspnea from chronic pulmonary disease, the extreme fatigue in advanced cardiac disease, pain in diabetic neuropathy, or cachexia in Human Immunodeficiency Virus (HIV) or Acquired Immune Deficiency Syndrome (AIDS). The common element across diseases and symptoms is that suffering is experienced by *people*, not bodily organs. That which threatens the wholeness or the survival of the person results in suffering.

Although there are common characteristics of suffering and similarities between individual experiences or disease contexts, there are also profound differences. One person's experience of a chronic illness may be characterized as mild disruption in life, whereas a person with a similar physical diagnosis may experience devastation, profound spiritual consequences, and intense suffering. There are many possible explanations for these varied responses, but one factor is a person's cultural context.

Culture significantly influences an individual's reaction to illness or disability. Culture provides the foundation for all life experiences and profoundly influences the response to illness. Cultures hold strong beliefs about illness. Culture influences how one responds to declining health or a new diagnosis, as well as to all aspects of treatment and the disease trajectory. Additionally, the capacity for patients to give meaning to suffering and transcend that suffering is intimately related to cultural beliefs and values (Chiu, 2000; Ferrell and Sun, 2006).

Culture is also closely bound in language and ritual. Understanding and respecting culturally held beliefs, customs, language, and rituals will enable nurses to gain a glimpse into the lens through which a patient views life. In assessing cultural influences on suffering, nurses may find it helpful to explore their own as well as their patients' past experiences with illness, to ask about the influence of religion and spirituality, and to gain insight into their interpretations of suffering, pain, and death.

THE NEED FOR A UNIQUE ANALYSIS OF NURSING AND SUFFERING

Nurses are the constant presence for patients and families as they experience illness across all settings of care. From the acute onset of illness or the moment of diagnosis of a chronic disease, individuals look to the face of a nurse for reassurance, understanding, and as a human connection in the overwhelming reality of health care.

In the United States, there are more than 2.8 million registered nurses. The experiences of these nurses who bear witness to suffering are a valuable voice to articulate lived experiences of people of all ages in their most vulnerable and broken states. Yet, the title of "nurse" is a broad category. These 2.8 million nurses include a spectrum of human beings as diverse as the patients they serve. A night-shift nurse caring for a seriously ill, distraught, and complex patient may be a 22-year-old new graduate, with limited nursing or life experience. Yet she is the professional on the front line, directing the care of a suffering patient. The day nurse who relieves this new graduate may be a 55-year-old man with 30 years of cumulative professional and personal experiences of triumph, loss, relieving pain, and witnessing suffering. He may also bring to the bedside his own intense personal experience of the recent deaths of his parents.

Although, as a profession, nursing is often recognized for addressing whole-person care, there are aspects of nursing that contradict the necessary response to suffering (Jackson, 2003). Nurses are often similar to physicians, guilty of a "fix-it" approach to care. We want to heal the wound, eliminate the pain, relieve the nausea, and increase function. Many nurses, the authors of this text included, were taught that a "good nurse" was one whose patients ate well and consumed sufficient fluids, had functioning bowels and bladders, breathed deeply, and ambulated independently—preferably by the end of the nurse's shift!

Our nursing education (and thus our journey to "becoming" nurses) was guided by a nursing process and a nursing care plan that often resembled a checklist of actions to restore the sick to health and the dependent to independence. Our educational preparation was void of philosophy, role modeling, or reward for behaviors such as compassion and presence. The concept of communication in nursing practice was reduced to "patient teaching" in which an informed nurse directed the uninformed patient toward restored health. Communication was not about the art of listening or witnessing suffering. Yet somewhere on the journey to our learning "healing" instead of "teaching," many of us had the profound gift of witnessing true nursing by a seasoned and compassionate colleague. Watching a nurse who is fully present, who listens carefully and says little but provides the sufferer the opportunity of "voice" as described by Reich (1987, 1989), is a true education. Such mentors teach us that silencing or stifling the voice of suffering serves only to intensify it.

The same nursing process that guides our "fix-it" philosophy can guide our response to suffering. Nurses *assess* patients to identify sources of unnecessary suffering, such as unrelieved pain or other symptoms, expressions of shame, or feelings of spiritual abandonment by a God who has allowed serious illness and "untimely" death. Nurses *diagnose* sources of suffering and identify those that can and should be relieved, and they recognize the aspects of illness and suffering that should be witnessed and supported.

Nurses *intervene* through presence, listening, and communication that enables patient expression and by eliminating sources of suffering such as pain. The nurse in the chemotherapy clinic informs the patient of the hair loss that will soon begin, offering a sense of control over a frequently devastating and terrifying bodily loss. On the next visit, the nurse listens carefully to the patient's story as she describes what it feels like to see more hair on the pillow than her head. The nurse understands the woman's decision to shave her head for a "fast torture" rather than "slow agony." The nurse offers a scarf or a wig, aware that it may never be worn but understanding that the gesture of offering a wig provides recognition that this nauseated, bald, anxious, weak patient is still a person and a woman and that her hair loss matters.

Nurses complete the nursing process through constant *evaluation*, ever vigilant about altering the plan of care, recognizing new problems, and meeting the patient's needs. Using these stages of the nursing process, the response to suffering then becomes a form of nursing that may not restore function or "fix" a problem but a form of nursing that helps to soothe wounded dignity and restore a sense of humanity.

Exploring the concept of suffering from the perspective of those who experience it and those who witness it is vital if we are to advance our care. Although research and literature is limited in relation to this common phenomenon of suffering, we do know that suffering extends beyond physical pain and represents a deeply personal state. Most of us have experienced suffering—to be human is to suffer. But unnecessary suffering is something different.

Researchers from Canada (Daneault, et al. 2004) explored the nature of suffering and its relief through a qualitative study of 26 terminally ill patients with cancer. Their findings revealed that patients experienced suffering in the dimensions of physical, psychological, and social well being. The content analysis of the interviews recognized what the researchers described as three irreducible, core dimensions of suffering: *(1)* being subjected to violence, *(2)* being deprived and overwhelmed, and *(3)* living in apprehension.

In a similar study, nurse researchers from Finland explored suffering in patients with advanced cancer (Kuuppalomaki and Sirkka, 1998). Their research found suffering to exist in the same three dimensions of physical, psychological, and social well being as recognized by the Canadian researchers. Physical suffering included fatigue, pain, and side effects of chemotherapy. Psychological suffering, most commonly expressed as depression, was related to the physical changes resulting from the disease and overall debilitation as death became imminent. The physical and psychological effects of the worsened disease caused withdrawal and isolation, hence the third dimension of spiritual suffering. This study reinforced the inter-relatedness of the dimensions of suffering and the whole-person phenomenon.

The findings of the Canadian and Finnish researchers were very similar to a study by a nurse researcher in the United States who studied suffering in patients with lung cancer (Benedict, 1989). It is interesting to note the similarities in these studies and the common descriptions of distress from patients across diverse countries and cultures. Studies such as these help us to understand patient experiences of suffering and to uncover sources of suffering.

Roberto Rodriguez is a 72-year-old homeless man living in San Diego, California. Having immigrated from Mexico 3 years ago, he came to a community clinic seeking relief from continuous pain, nausea, and diarrhea associated with advanced pancreatic cancer. Roberto came to California 1 year ago at the urging of his son, a dock worker in a shipyard. Shortly after Roberto arrived, his son was killed in an accident.

Roberto is a quiet, stoic man who graciously accepts any relief the clinic can provide. Over the past 4 months, he has been seen regularly by James, a clinic nurse. Roberto is self-conscious of his appearance, his social situation as a homeless man, and his increasing reliance on the clinic as his body declines. In recent visits, Roberto has started to express his suffering to James as he speaks of his elderly mother left behind in Mexico, the wife he abandoned a year ago at the height of his alcoholism, the painful loss of his son, and his worsening symptoms.

James has worked diligently with the clinic social worker to maximize all possible care for Roberto. He refers to the patient always as Mr. Rodriguez, and acknowledges his kindness to the other clinic patients and his willingness to wait as sicker patients are seen first. James has encouraged Roberto to take his pain medication, assuring him that his use of the morphine is not addiction. Today, James discreetly provided Roberto with adult diapers to wear when his diarrhea becomes extreme.

James' goal is to see Roberto placed in a long-term care setting for what likely will be only a few weeks to months of remaining life. He and the clinic staff are desperately working to achieve placement amidst a bureaucratic, overburdened, inefficient county health-care system that has lost their request and seems unlikely to respond in time. James' hope is that Roberto will not die alone and that his symptoms will be relieved. This week, James arranged for a volunteer Catholic chaplain to be present at the time of Roberto's visit and orchestrated a private encounter in a clinic room while Roberto awaited the physician visit.

Roberto tells the chaplain that James has been "the face of God" and that if not for James, he would not come to the clinic. Roberto asks the chaplain for one favor: When he is "no longer coming to the clinic" the chaplain should give James a tarnished metal cross he carries in his pocket.

James' care for Roberto is symbolic of the nursing response to the suffering of strangers. His greatest service is his presence. He listens to the losses of this man's life, offering unconditional support, attention to his dignity, relief of physical symptoms, and advocacy for health-care resources. James is a personal link to an overwhelming, bureaucratic system. He is concerned with Roberto's physical pain and his privately expressed suffering.

One of the major contributions to nursing scholarship in the area of suffering is the work of Kahn and Steeves (1996), who described the basic tenets of suffering. These scholars defined the nurse as a witness and moral agent. They described a witness as a special kind of moral agent with an obligation to speak out about what is witnessed. The authors encouraged "speaking out" and the development of nursing's collective voice in response to suffering.

The role of witness is described by Kahn and Steeves in four ways. In *firsthand observations*, nurses are closest to the patient and have an opportunity to inform others about what has been observed. *Ceremonial role* occurs when nurses reduce suffering by supporting or participating in rituals of transition or "rites of passage" that require witnesses to substantiate them. An *expert witness* is one who testifies or speaks in public forums about the special knowledge his or her expertise brings to a public issue. Nurses have spoken out in their own institutions and, increasingly, in public forums about issues such as unrelieved pain, grief, and loss. The *visionary* role is one in which nursing's collective vision develops as each nurse speaks out about the suffering he or she encounters, how best to respond to it, and the need for a future in which suffering is not ignored. Visionary nurses are currently challenging the care provided in settings such as neonatal ICU (NICU), homeless communities, and psychiatric care.

Box 1.1. Tenets of Suffering As Described by Kahn and Steeves (1996)

- Suffering is a private, lived experience of a whole person, unique to each individual.
- Suffering results when the most important aspects of a person's identity are threatened or lost.
- Because suffering depends on the meaning of an event or loss for the individual, it cannot be assumed present or absent in any given clinical condition.
- Suffering also can be viewed as an experience of lost personal meaning.
- Possible sources of suffering are innumerable.
- We recognize certain kinds of experiences as forms of suffering; we acknowledge these forms as experiences that will lead to suffering for many who experience them.
- As a fundamental human experience, suffering has a basic structure.
- The experience of suffering involves the person in a larger process that includes the person's own coping with suffering and the caring of others.
- The caring environment in which the processes of suffering occur can influence a person's suffering positively and negatively.

Box 1.1. presents the tenets of suffering described by Kahn and Steeves. The unique voice of nursing in exploration of suffering is evident in this work. The last tenet, which states that suffering can be influenced by the caring environment, is the call to action for nurses.

OVERVIEW OF THE CONTENT AND APPROACH TO THIS BOOK

As the authors of this text, we are interested in giving voice to the nature of suffering and the goals of nursing through sharing our own thoughts and career observations. This work is intended as a nursing voice, both in the description of patient suffering and in the description of nurses' responses. Although we have attempted to represent a spectrum of patient and nurse experiences, this work is certainly biased toward chronic and terminal illness and is strongly influenced by our focus on oncology. While we acknowledge the tremendous diversity of nursing and of patients, we believe many common elements exist, irrespective of this diversity in patients and nurses. We are all, at the core, human beings experiencing illness or responding to suffering. The similarities between an emergency room nurse comforting a 30-year-old man in sickle cell crisis and an oncology clinic nurse administering the first dose of chemotherapy to a terrified 60-year-old woman newly diagnosed with breast cancer are enormous. The human suffering is more similar than different.

The book is the culmination of more than 70 years of nursing experience of the authors. Nessa Coyle, Ph.D., NP., is a nurse at Memorial Sloan Kettering Cancer Center in New York and was co-editor (with Betty Ferrell, Ph.D., R.N.) of *The Textbook of Palliative Nursing*, also published by Oxford University Press. In 2004, Betty Ferrell returned to graduate school at Claremont Graduate University to complete a Master's degree in Theology, Ethics, and Culture. During that period, Nessa Coyle completed a 1-year postgraduate course in Bioethics and Medical Humanities offered through Montefiore Medical Center/Albert Einstein College of Medicine and Cardoza Law School in New York City. Our intent is to complement our co-edited *Textbook of Palliative Nursing*, which focuses largely on the science of palliative nursing, with this book, which captures the art of nursing as a caring profession responding to suffering.

Chapter 2 of this book, "Ethical and Theological Perspectives on the Nature of Suffering and the Goals of Nursing," is an attempt to move beyond nursing or medical literature to apply knowledge from fields such as feminist ethics, spirituality, and theology to examine the concept of suffering.

Chapter 3 is "A Contextual Analysis of Suffering." This chapter intends to bring the suffering person's voice to this text. The perspectives include those of pediatrics, critical care, oncology, geriatrics, pain management, and family caregivers. These contexts were selected as clinical areas recognized as places of pervasive suffering and those with intense nursing involvement. The suffering seen in these settings is described in this chapter by nurses who have witnessed the suffering within these contexts.

Bearing witness to suffering across these contexts exacts a toll on the witness—the nurse. Therefore, Chapter 4, "Contextual Analysis of Nurses' Own Suffering," is a discussion of nurses' own suffering. This chapter explores the topic of the moral distress of nurses who witness futile care. It also discusses the distress and conflict nurses feel in inflicting "necessary" pain while providing care. As this chapter illustrates, technological advances in care have created a health-care system that often seeks to prolong life with consequences of greatly diminished QOL and moral distress to nurses on the front lines of care. Nurses, like patients, are first and foremost people. The professional work of nursing requires boundaries, self-knowledge, and personal awareness of one's own attitudes and feelings about the meaning of life and of death. Failure to care for oneself ultimately diminishes the ability of the nurse to witness or relieve the suffering of patients or their families. This last sentence could be written in bold at the beginning and end of every chapter. Providing care for others without caring for oneself is unsustainable.

Chapter 5 of the book is, "Toward a Model of the Nature of Suffering and the Goals of Nursing." Because we begin this text with a discussion of the deficiencies in current models to describe suffering from a nursing perspective, we end it with a synthesis of clinical experiences and narratives from nurses and patients to offer a perspective on suffering that more closely captures the essence of nursing. We conclude with recommendations for nursing as we continue to care for those who suffer in a system that is chaotic and troubled.

There are three sources of data that have informed this text. The first has been descriptions of suffering as derived from the literature. The literature reviewed has been selected based on searches of medical, nursing, ethics, theology, and other literature. For the thesis, the focus has been on literature with the greatest clinical application. All of the literature cited in the references has been cited in the text. Hundreds of additional citations were reviewed but those included reflect literature that was felt to be most clinically relevant to suffering associated with illness.

The second source of data that has informed this work has been narrative data derived from interviews or written comments from patients, family caregivers, and nurses. These data were abstracted from several studies we conducted and analyzed. For the purpose of this work, the data were re-evaluated from the perspective of suffering. Narrative data were also collected from the ELNEC courses, which had not been analyzed. Narrative data were interpreted using content analysis methods. The narratives of nurses, patients, and family members have been analyzed to identify common themes and concepts related to suffering. In the concluding section of Chapter 3, we move beyond individual contexts of suffering to describe the essence of suffering from a nursing perspective.

The third source of information for this work has been our personal and professional experiences. Beverly Harrison (1985) and Carol Gilligan (1982), as well as many other feminist scholars, have acknowledged that personal reflection and narrative is a valued source of scholarship. The case examples included in these chapters are based on actual patients cared for by the authors or have been shared with them by nursing colleagues and have been edited to emphasize aspects of suffering and to ensure anonymity. To embrace the depths of suffering requires scholarly inquiry, synthesis of the literature, and reflection on clinical experiences and the lived observations of those who suffer.

Chapters 1–3 were completed by capturing patient and family narratives, and Chapter 4 was developed to describe the nurse's own suffering. After completion of these four chapters, we took a step back and looked at the whole to identify the nature of suffering from this analysis. A list of key themes from Chapters 1–4 was created (Table 5.1 in Chapter 5) and was then reviewed and synthesized to conclude this text. The concluding chapter is an attempt to distill the essence of the nature of suffering and the goals of nursing.

THE UNIQUE RELATIONSHIP OF THE PATIENT AND NURSE

While many health-care professionals are involved with patients' suffering from illness, this text addresses the unique relationship of the patient and nurse. The features of this relationship are illustrated in the following case.

❧

Mrs. Marietta Krakaski is a 78-year-old Polish woman currently hospitalized after experiencing a stroke. She has responded well to the acute care received in the emergency department and ICU and is now on the neurology floor of an academic medical center. She is being seen by four medical specialties, as well as speech therapy, physical

*therapy, and occupational therapy. Now that she is stable, she is un-
dergoing further diagnostic work to evaluate her cardiovascular status
and to determine her overall health status in planning her post-stroke
rehabilitation. She has short-term memory loss, unsteady gait, elevated
blood pressure, and some left-sided weakness as well as expressive
aphasia.*

*During the night shift, after a day that has included encounters
with no less than 20 different health-care professionals, attendants,
transporters, and visitors, Mrs. Krakaski is found sobbing quietly by
the night nurse who has entered to check her telemetry. She denies pain
but admits that the reality of the stroke "just hit me." She tearfully
speaks for a few moments with the nurse, who softly strokes her hand
and offers a tissue. As their eyes connect, Mrs. Krakaski's quiet sobs
become intense and she clutches the nurse's hand, repeating intensely
"I have to get well . . . I have to get well."*

*After finally calming her, the nurse asks her to try to explain her
fears and to specifically express her greatest concern. Mrs. Krakaski
says that she must return home soon, this week, as she is the only
caregiver for her elderly husband who has advanced prostate cancer.
She shares that their son has come from another state but can only stay
a few days and that he and his father don't get along, thus she is
worried about what may be happening at home. She tells the nurse that
she has promised to be there for her husband because he has always
been there for her, including a few years ago when she was treated for
breast cancer. She also shares that her 50-year-old daughter died of
breast cancer last year.*

*Mrs. Krakaski asks the nurse to please try to convince the doctors
to let her go home. She also tells the nurse that if a priest is ever in the
hospital at night, she would like to see him. She explains that she can't
ask for a priest during the daytime when her husband might be visiting
because he "no longer believes there can be a God."*

The case of Marietta Krakaski and the nighttime encounter with a nurse
illustrates the unique place of nursing amidst a complex health-care system.
Marietta is surrounded by many caregivers, yet it is within an intimate,
personal encounter with a nurse that her suffering is expressed. In the
darkness of her room the patient shares her greatest fears, life losses, and her
request for help, and she exposes her vulnerability as her physical body
forces her to become a "patient," thus betraying her role as "caregiver" for
her spouse. The nurse becomes her confidant, the vessel of her anxiety, and
the counselor for her spiritual distress.

SUMMARY

We have been inspired by Cassell's 1982 work on the nature of suffering and the goals of medicine. His work provides a foundation for the exploration of nurses' voice in describing the nature of suffering and in articulating the goals of nursing. We communicated our intent to write this parallel analysis for nursing with Dr. Cassell and his gracious, enthusiastic response was a valued source of encouragement. We thank him for starting this conversation, now exactly 25 years ago. We are honored to now articulate a nursing voice.

Witnessing suffering is the everyday work of nurses. In every setting, across diseases, and in people of all ages, suffering is part of being human, often intensified when being human also involves being ill. This work is intended as a step toward supporting nurses who care constantly for those who suffer. Kahn and Steeves (1994) captured the intent of this work in writing: "One characteristic of nursing's development over the past decade is the discovery of its voice—the ability and willingness to express what nurses collectively know and understand about the nature of nursing practice. To continue the development of nursing's voice, it is crucial that we talk freely about what we know, including what we know about suffering."

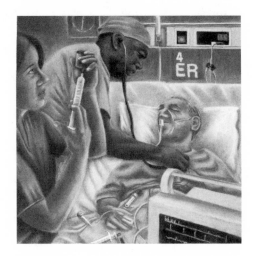

CHAPTER 2 ☙

Ethical and Theological Perspectives on the Nature of Suffering and the Goals of Nursing

Chapter 1 presented an overview of thoughts related to suffering derived from the medical and nursing literature and experience. In this chapter, we apply scholarly work from the fields of theology and ethics to provide a different perspective on suffering. The chapter begins with a foundational exploration of the limits to current approaches to suffering and then explores ethical perspectives followed by theological perspectives. Within the theological perspective, we explore the concept of forgiveness to show that the depth of understanding of suffering available in this field can be applied to the nursing perspective. We also follow with a discussion of meeting diverse religious beliefs with particular concern for nursing amidst our increasingly diverse society.

LIMITS OF CURRENT APPROACHES TO SUFFERING

The profession of nursing shares many characteristics with the medical profession. This is not surprising because, until relatively recently, the nursing curriculum has paralleled that of medicine. Although nurses have always been educated separately, the early focus of nursing education was on nurses following medical orders. Both disciplines focus on goals of cure, rehabilitation, restoration, and optimizing function. Both fields are often characterized by a "fix-it" approach, where a professional makes a diagnosis and then "fixes" the broken body part, organ, or function.

From the earliest clinical experiences as nursing students, we are rewarded for our skill at identifying problems and solving them. We move the patient from dependence to independence, from brokenness to wholeness. Nurses are "doers;" our work is in doing procedures, medicating, teaching, ambulating, documenting, and communicating. We also have been taught to be listeners and mediators as we bridge communication among patients, families, and multiple clinical personnel. Given this historical and educational foundation of "doing" and "fixing" and "mediating," it is not surprising that so few nurses feel comfortable and competent to "be with" a person who is suffering. The ability to "be with" suffering and bear with the sufferer is an art, generally mastered after extensive life experience, self-reflection, and concentrated professional development (Dahlin and Giansiracusa, 2006).

The deficiencies in our collective nursing ability to respond to suffering can be seen in our approach to the assessment of spirituality. In our increasingly diverse culture, we are called to recognize that spirituality is a broad term. For our purposes, we use the definition of spirituality as the "transcendent dimension of life which extends beyond organized religion" (Kemp, 2006). The basic spiritual needs include seeking meaning or purpose, hope, relatedness, forgiveness or acceptance, and transcendence (Kemp, 2006).

Even in major health-care settings, assessment of spirituality is often limited to a brief question on a hospital admission form of religion, generally followed by a short list of choices such as Protestant, Catholic, Jewish, or "Other." Our systems of care, with a few exceptions, even for those facing life-threatening disease, rarely explores any aspect of spirituality, meaning, and relationship to God or a higher power or the importance of faith (Borneman and Brown-Saltzman, 2006).

ETHICAL PERSPECTIVES ON SUFFERING IN NURSING

The phenomenon of *presence*, which is so central to nursing, was described poignantly by theologian and ethicist William Reich (1987, 1989). Reich described the experience of suffering through the metaphor of language. He described the person's struggle to discover a voice in the search for the meaning of suffering, divided into three phases. These include mute suffering, expressive suffering, and new identity.

In mute suffering, patients are so affected by their circumstances that they cannot verbally express their needs. This is not "suffering in silence," because Reich asserted that these individuals may be "screaming in pain." In expressive suffering, the sufferer seeks a language. The language may be one of lament (complaint), storytelling (in telling their story they gain voice, transform the suffering, or gain distance), or interpretation (often through metaphor). The third phase is new identity, or having a voice of one's own. This occurs through experiencing solidarity with compassionate others and by taking on a language of suffering through reframing one's story, which then identifies the new self. Reich's work can be aptly applied to the compassionate work of nurses who respond to the "screams of pain" by patients who only appear to "suffer in silence" (Reich, 1987, 1989).

Similar to the concentration placed on cure or "fixing," medical and nursing orientation to ethics is also often narrowly focused. We have given predominant attention in our training, coursework, and clinical ethics consultation to a biomedical model. The principles of autonomy, beneficence, nonmalfeasance, and justice serve as the primary approach to virtually all ethical dilemmas (Stanley and Zoloth-Dorfman, 2006). However, there are nursing educational programs and ethics committees that have recognized other frameworks and approaches to clinical dilemmas. The contribution of feminist scholarship offers a valuable alternate lens for nursing with an emphasis on concepts such as care, respect, and compassion (Farley, 1990; Procter-Smith, 1995; Townes, 1995) in addition to autonomy and beneficence.

The following is a case example of the complex needs inherent in a clinical dilemma.

An 86-year-old man is admitted to the hospital after a fall in a nursing home, which fractured his hip. Following his hip pinning, the man continues to experience complications of anesthesia and unrelieved pain, resulting in sleep deprivation with subsequent confusion, urinary incontinence, and a wound infection. His son arrives from out of town and is distraught at seeing his father, whom he has not seen in months. He expresses his remorse at "putting my dad in a damn nursing home." When the patient continues to decline and develops pneumonia and an arrythmia, the son elects to "do it all," requesting a feeding tube, mechanical ventilation, tracheostomy, and transfer to another hospital "if you idiots who are killing my father can't turn this around." This request comes despite a completed advanced directive on record in which the father has clearly indicated he wants no life-prolonging treatments. The son insists his father wouldn't need his life prolonged were it not for the "idiots" in the nursing home who let him fall and the hospital "idiots" who made him worse.

Resolution of this complex, but not uncommon, scenario requires more than a matter of ethical principles, laws, forms, procedures, or blame. It requires allowing a process to unfold embracing the concepts of care, compassion, and respect. This includes listening to the son's story as he gives voice to his suffering and frustration at the same time as respecting the dignity and advance directives of his father.

Ethical approaches based on the concept of care provide a framework for transcending a place of obligation (what we ought to do based on laws or professional standards) so we can determine our moral obligation as compassionate witnesses. Dr. Daniel Sulmasy, a physician and Franciscan Friar, has been a thoughtful contributor to the evolving understanding of the professional as healer in relationship with the sufferer (Sulmasy, 2006). Sulmasy wrote *The Rebirth of the Clinic: An Introduction to Spirituality in Health Care*, in which he challenges the medical profession to evaluate itself and to restore a sense of the sacred to health care. He cites Jewish philosopher and theologian Abraham Heschel (1955), who said "To heal a person, one must first be a person." Awareness of one's own spirituality may be one prerequisite to ethical behavior and to meeting the challenge posed by Sulmasy to treat all patients as people first.

Sulmasy's challenge to reform the "clinic" is directed toward physicians, as "spiritual–scientific practitioners," but his work has profound implications for nurses. As we advance the education and research of our profession, we are challenged to also advance our understanding and clinical competence in aspects of spirituality. Sulmasy wrote:

> Under this new medical covenant, a spiritual-scientific practitioner would affirm that the transcendent is made manifest at the edge of the surgeon's knife, at the tips of the palpating fingers of the pediatrician, in the firm handshake of the internist, in the birth of the child whose unwed mother has AIDS, in the tears of the woman who feels a hard lump in her one remaining breast, and in the vacant stare of the elderly man with dementia. A spiritual-scientific practitioner would affirm that the transcendent is there when disease and suffering are recognized together, when the hand that performs the spinal tap distills compassion into the needle's point, the objectivity of science with the subjectivity of God's healing will; the particularity of the case at hand with the universality of a profession under oath; the finitude of the moment and the infinity of a life lived in the service of love. Thus might the clinic be reborn. (Sulmasy, 2006, 85)

What will it take to instill the sacred to nursing? Most would agree that the state of health care is chaotic at best. In some settings, it is disastrous. Instilling a sense of the sacred is a big step for a nurse who is focused on survival: both her patients' and her own. Patient acuity is at an all-time high. The nursing shortage grows. With all these issues, how can we even consider suffering? Perhaps more importantly, how can we not?

Caring for the dying is only one of nursing's many challenges for alleviating suffering. Nurses care for countless patients who suffer from chronic illness and are not considered "terminal." However, tending to those who are dying allows nurses to reflect on the sacred nature of their work as they witness both despair and transcendence in others. As Sulmasy wrote:

> The dying person brings his or her entire life to the moment of death. Christian theology teaches that if a life has the love of the Incarnate God as the foundation of its value, the source of its hope, and its model of right relationship, this trinity of value, hope, and right relationship is exactly what will be irrevocably, absolutely, and eternally determined in the dying of that person. Caring for a patient who is dying in such a manner is a remarkable privilege. When I enter the room of such a patient (which happens far more often than those who do not care for dying persons might think), I sometimes wonder if I should remove my shoes because I know that the ground on which I am about to tread is holy. I find that I am the one transformed, the one to whom enormous grace has been revealed. Such an experience is more than enough to sustain a doctor or nurse in hospice or palliative care. It is grace enough for the dying. (Sulmasy, 2006, 212)

This grace is perhaps why nurses are drawn to the bedside of a patient who is "dying well." Such a person expresses wonder and awe in what they see unfolding before them. The nurse might be mystified about how this person seems so accepting and peaceful, when so many others die in such anguish. Why is this death different? Nurses not infrequently stand at the foot of a bed watching as a patient takes his last breath. Where has the life force gone? Where has the person gone? The man or woman who was here before us just a moment ago is gone and what is left is a body vacant of life. What has the nurse witnessed?

THEOLOGICAL PERSPECTIVES

Nurses, as the intimate caregivers of those who suffer, are often confronted by questions such as, "Why does my father have to suffer?" "What did I do to deserve this?" "How can God cause my mother such pain?" The questioning of God and the search for meaning in overwhelming situations of illness is equaled and often surpassed by family and friends who witness the patient suffering. The suffering of a spouse is described here.

I am the husband of a patient in pain. My wife has been diagnosed with a disease but it is the devastation of that disease that we live each day. I am my wife's support, her cheerleader, her shoulder, her hope. I put on a deceiving face of hope and smile. And yet, my spirit could not feel more depleted. In my life at work, I control 100 people, and yet at the end of the day I return to my home, which is controlled by pain. How much can you watch; how long can you endure the face of pain? I am walking a tightrope. One in which my daily wish is for the nightmare to end and for my wife's disease to be better. Between those hopes, I occasionally allow myself to face an unspoken wish that if she cannot be cured of this disease, must she be made to live with this unrelenting pain? Bearing witness to illness is one thing. Bearing witness to pain is quite another . . . I, too, cannot sleep. I am anxious and depressed and fearful. I am attempting to be provider, spouse, father, and mother. I turn to my fragile and damaged life partner seeking intimacy and find an even more frail and delicate person than I have recognized. Amidst my myriad of roles, I am now asked to be the primary care provider for my wife in the home . . . As I measure medication, I shudder at the reality that I am pouring a dose of morphine for my wife. Am I delivering mercy? Relief? Should I be fearful of these medications? Am I doing harm? There is something surreal about this way of being that now fills my daily life. I am not the patient in pain. I am the witness. (Ferrell, 2005)

Watching the suffering of the loved ones of patients can create an additional burden for nurses to carry, especially if they are unschooled and unprepared in how to "work with" this suffering.

In a pediatric oncology unit, a mother comforts a young child undergoing a bone marrow biopsy for relapsed leukemia. After hours of holding and comforting a bald, cachectic, bruised, and exhausted child, the father arrives to offer respite, and the mother retreats to the nurses' station. She asks for a cup of coffee. As the nurse hands the mother the coffee, there is a connection: first of hands, then eyes and hearts. Without a spoken word, the mother cries, releasing the burden of the last few hours. The nurse offers a tissue and a chair. More importantly, she offers an acknowledgement of the suffering with her presence, the presence of a person unafraid to listen. Questions such as, "How can this be?" "How much more can he take?" "Isn't there an easier way?" are common. So is anger. The overwhelmed mother asks, "Why can't I be the one who is sick, not him?" She tells the nurse, "When I get to heaven, there's going to be some serious conversation between me and God."

Some scholars have described suffering as "spiritual pain" (Chochinov, 2006). Suffering is described as an existential crisis and loss of meaning. Suffering at the end of life commonly includes hopelessness, a feeling of being a burden to others, loss of dignity, and the will to live (Chochinov, 2006).

In a recent text titled *Health and Human Flourishing—Religion, Medicine, and Moral Anthropology*, the authors (Taylor and Dell'Oro, 2006) cited Scheler's statement that, "In the ten thousand years of history, we are the first age in which man has become utterly and unconditionally problematic to himself in which he no longer knows who he is, but at the same time knows he does not know" (Scheler, 1962). Taylor and Dell'Oro conclude by saying that in the twenty-first century, we know much about man as a biological being but not as much about who, what, or why he is and that, "without a clearer idea of what man is, we will enter and remain in a dark moral forest without a compass" (Taylor and Dell'Oro, 2006, 267). A deeper understanding of suffering may provide that moral compass, giving us both values as well as direction and the opportunity for daily practice.

The writings of French philosopher and mystic Simone Weil (Springstead, 1998) and German theologian Dorothee Soelle (1975) are relevant sources to support the compass that can guide nurses' understanding of suffering. Weil wrote of suffering in her treatise on "The Love of God and Affliction." She converted from agnosticism to Christianity and wrote from her personal experiences with tuberculosis and anorexia. These diseases ended her life in early adulthood. Weil distinguished physical pain from suffering. She said that pain is of "little account" and that "an hour or two of violent pain caused by a bad tooth is nothing once it is over" (Springstead, 1998, 42). Weil described "affliction" as "suffering." Worse than affliction, she said, is extreme affliction. "Extreme affliction means physical pain, distress of soul and social degradation, all together, is the nail. The point of the nail is applied to the very center of the soul, and its head is the whole of necessity throughout all space and time" (Springstead, 1998, 54).

William Reich, a theologian cited previously for his comments on mute suffering, also wrote on the subject of compassion. He said that examination of compassion must begin with an understanding of suffering because the need for compassion is created by suffering, not just by pain. He further defined suffering as "an anguish we experience on one level as a threat to our composure, our integrity, and the fulfillment of our intentions but at a deeper level as a frustration to the concrete meaning that we have found in our personal existence" (Reich, 1989, 85).

Similar to the phases of suffering previously described, Reich also identified three phases of compassion (Reich, 1989). The first phase is silent empathy/silent compassion. In this phase, the caregiver is silent in witnessing the suffering of another. The second phase is expressive compassion in which caregivers help to "give voice to the voiceless" by listening to their stories and helping convert the sufferers' experiences into comprehensible words. The final phase is a compassionate voice of one's own. In this phase, the compassionate caregiver is also transformed by witnessing the suffering of another and by making systematic changes to relieve the suffering.

Reich's phases of compassion can be applied to nursing. A neonatal nurse has worked for several years in an inner city NICU, listening with compassion to the tears and voices of young parents whose preterm infants have died despite the high-tech heroic efforts of neonatal care. The nurse is distraught in knowing that these parents leave the hospital with no follow-up, no money for funeral costs, and no access to counseling or bereavement services. The nurse appeals to hospital administration, sharing years of her observations of these dying babies and their parents, giving voice to the inadequate system that ignores their suffering during the NICU stay and after death.

The nurse's own suffering, and that of her colleagues, is diminished as they are successful in changing the system of care. Despite the desperate lack of resources, the hospital arranges for a psychology intern placement and part-time chaplain for the unit. A referral arrangement is made for bereavement support in the local mental health clinic. The nurses establish a routine of sending bereavement cards to parents and an annual memorial service is established. The infants, their parents, and the nurses now experience a transformed system responsive to suffering.

Similarly to the writings of Reich, McGrath (2002) described spiritual pain as a sense of diffuse emotional and existential pain related to meaninglessness and pain resulting from a break with usual relationships that connect one to life. Spiritual pain and suffering are often described in terms of despair, depression, request for hastened death, and hopelessness

(McClain-Jacobson, et al. 2004; Ersek, 2006). People facing chronic disabling illness or those at life's end often become overwhelmed with the burdens of daily life and the recognition of the burden of their life on others.

There is growing consensus regarding the key factors influencing psychological and spiritual well-being in terminal illness. Lin and Bauer-Wu (2003) conducted an extensive literature review and concluded that key factors in psychospiritual coping included self-awareness, coping and adjusting to stress, relationships/connections to others, faith, a sense of empowerment and confidence, and living with meaning and hope.

Another model of care responsive to suffering has been work by Chochinov (2006), who has developed a psychotherapy program titled "Dignity Therapy," which integrates spiritual issues and resources for people with cancer. The four concerns of the program content are: control, identity, relationships, and meaning (Chochinov, 2006). Breitbart (2002) has conducted similar work in testing a "meaning-making intervention," which builds on classic work by Victor Frankl (1963). Frankl described the devastation of suffering that splits the whole person into fragments. He suggested that people are destroyed not by suffering itself but by suffering that is void of meaning. The intent of both these therapies is to increase the sense of meaning, dignity, and hopefulness in the face of serious illness or other devastating circumstances.

A CASE ILLUSTRATION OF FORGIVENESS

The concept of forgiveness serves as an excellent example of the relevance of theology to the clinical care of patients at the end of life. Individuals facing death often reflect on their lives and relationships and confront unresolved conflicts from the past. The following case illustrates this topic.

Mr. Farber is a 60-year-old Jewish man who, with his young family, moved from Israel to America 30 years ago. He was first a bookkeeper and, after many years of evening classes, became an accountant. He has worked hard to provide for his wife and five children. His wife is diabetic and has had many physical complications over the years. Mr. Farber is a loving husband and has nurtured his children, their spouses, and his grandchildren throughout their lives. Four months ago Mr. Farber was diagnosed with pancreatic cancer and more recently developed extensive brain metastasis. Two weeks ago he developed seizures, which was the final breaking point for his wife, who has tried desperately to care for him at home.

Now a patient in an inpatient hospice setting, Mr. Farber is visited by his entire family. The evening nurse is moved by this kind man. She finds herself touched by his gentle manner and his overt expressions of love for his family. His hospice room is covered with family portraits, albums filled with family vacation photos, cards made by grand-children, and several books on Judaism. Before the family leaves for the evening, they join hands and surround the bed, praying together that God will be with him through the night and offering thanks for their blessing of family.

After the family goes home, the nurse returns to Mr. Farber's room. She feels intuitively that there is something he is concerned about that may be preventing him from being at peace. She begins to talk with him and comment on his wonderful family. When Mr. Farber becomes quiet, the nurse sits quietly by the bedside. After a few moments, tears come to Mr. Farber's eyes. The nurse asks, "Mr. Farber, is there some-thing bothering you, something I can help with?" His tears continue and he says simply, "I am not a good man."

The nurse is surprised by the contrast between his words and her image of this gentle, loving father, spouse, and grandfather. He repeats the words, "I am not a good man," and then tells the nurse about how he had an argument with a brother over 30 years ago, and now, despite his brother's pleas, he has refused to reconcile with him. Mr. Farber openly sobs, telling the nurse how sorry he is that he has never forgiven his brother and how he hopes that his brother can forgive him after his death.

The above case illustrates a scenario of a patient seeking forgiveness through dialogue with a nurse. This is not unusual; however, hospice and palliative care literature has often addressed such a request for forgiveness as a simple process: the patient expresses regret, and the professional listens to the request, offers consultation, and then facilitates the patient in seeking forgiveness through saying, "I'm sorry." The person who has been offended accepts the apology. All is forgiven. The life-long burden is relieved in a few hours, or perhaps a few minutes. We fix things.

Review of theological literature suggests that the process of forgiveness is seldom this simple. An illustrative citation is the work by Ashby (2003), "Being Forgiven: Toward a Thicker Description of Forgiveness." Ashby (2003) builds on other theological works (Enright and Coyle, 1998; Alken, 1997; Muller-Fahrenholz, 1997; McCullough, Pargament, and Thoreson, 2000) that have explored forgiveness at a much deeper level.

These theologians emphasize a forgiveness that goes beyond a simple act of pardoning, excusing, forgetting, or denying (Ashby, 2003). Ashby wrote of a parallel process in which one person seeks forgiveness and one grants forgiveness. Ashby wrote of the "being forgiven" process as an intricate work that includes the injured party being open to offering that forgiveness. The injured person accepts and bears the pain of the insult and thus develops compassion for the offender. The injured person finds deep meaning in the suffering associated with the injury. Ashby (2003) and Enright and Coyle (1998) have suggested that the act of seeking forgiveness may go even deeper when the offender also seeks self-forgiveness.

Keeping these levels of forgiveness in mind, we can see that Mr. Farber's confession will not be reconciled by simple assurance by the nurse that he is a "good man." The depth of his suffering will also not likely be resolved in the next few moments or even by a simple "fix" such as an offer by the nurse to contact the brother or to assist the patient in writing a note to his estranged brother. Forgiveness that offers relief for long-held suffering might best be facilitated through a more intricate process, even in the face of impending death. The nurse may also be most effective when acting as a partner in an interdisciplinary team that includes a chaplain (in this case, a rabbi) and social worker, whose collective efforts can best facilitate the process of forgiveness. In the end, it is an intensely personal act for Mr. Farber to forgive himself or to seek forgiveness. The nurse may offer presence and serve as a confessional source for the patient. The nurse's very presence offers acceptance of the injury, and with that acceptance may come relief of suffering or self-forgiveness. Few words on the nurse's part need be spoken.

RECOGNITION OF DIVERSE RELIGIOUS AND SPIRITUAL BELIEFS

Another critical concern for nursing is learning to respond to the diversity in cultures and faith traditions among patients. Health professionals often have little competence in spiritual assessment or intervention, and their skill is often limited to responding to those whose religion is the same as their own. The following case illustrates the need for competence in addressing diverse spiritual needs.

Ernest Littlejohn is a 78-year-old Native American recently diagnosed with lung cancer. Mr. Littlejohn has lived his life on an Arizona reservation and reluctantly moved to Los Angeles 2 months ago to live with his son Edward. Mr. Littlejohn's wife died 3 years ago from diabetic complications. Neither of Edward's parents have used health-care services beyond the Native American healer. Despite his declining condition, Mr. Littlejohn has refused to seek health care; however, over the past week, he has experienced increased dyspnea and has now come to the emergency room (ER). An X-ray in the ER identified a large mass in his right lung, presumed to be a tumor. He reluctantly agrees to be admitted if his breathing can be relieved but says he wants no medical treatment for "whatever you find on those tests."

Over the following 3 days, the doctors confirm a diagnosis of ad-vanced lung cancer. Mr. Littlejohn's symptoms are improved with ox-ygen, morphine, and antibiotics, and he is now calm and comfortable. He is adamant about going home by morning. The nurses have ob-served that although Mr. Littlejohn has improved over the last 3 days, his son Edward and his daughter Gloria (who arrived from New Mexico) have become extremely anxious.

Overhearing a conversation at the nurses' station, a hospital or-derly tells the nurses that he may know why the son is anxious. The orderly shares that yesterday he was talking with Edward in Radiology after transporting Mr. Littlejohn for an X-ray. The orderly and Edward began to discuss their shared experiences of caring for ill parents. Ed-ward is worried that his father will kill himself once he is discharged. Two of his uncles have killed themselves after becoming ill. Edward told the orderly, "My father will not want to be a burden. He will want to honor his heritage and dignity."

The nurses responsible for Mr. Littlejohn want to offer compassionate, respectful, competent, and culturally sensitive care. Although the afore-mentioned case does not mention an organized religion, it is rich in factors related to the meaning of health and illness, beliefs about life and death, and issues regarding relationships between a son and father as well as among professionals, families, and patients. It also offers the opportunity for self-evaluation of health beliefs by the providers of care.

While knowledge of diverse religious traditions and beliefs is important, it is also helpful for nurses to recognize diverse perspectives on suffering (Puchalski, Dorff, and Hendi, 2004; Kemp, 2006). Nurses can do much to support spiritual care of patients and families. Exploring the patient's spir-itual history, cultural beliefs, family traditions, and prayers can create a foun-dation for respecting and supporting spiritual needs (Fox, 2001).

People who hold Christian beliefs may see suffering through the life and death of Jesus Christ. People who are Catholic or Protestant may see suf-fering as an experience of being "with Christ"—as Christ suffered, so I suffer. Suffering may mean that the soul is tested, sins are forgiven, and redemption is gained. As a case example, a mother of a young adolescent boy dying from sarcoma refused pain medications for her son, despite his agonizing bone pain. This illustrative case follows.

The mother was not evil or "crazy" but she explains that her son had been in a gang and had never been "saved." She hopes his suffering would bring him close to God, and she also explains that pain medicine makes him sleepy and that it was important to keep him awake so that she could pray with him. When a well-intentioned home-care nurse asks the mother how she can stand to see her son spend his last days in pain, the mother becomes very angry. "You nurses think you care more about my son than I do. You are worried about a few days. I am worried about his eternal life." Fortunately, through expert and sensitive efforts by the nurse, chaplain, and a social worker, the mother was able to agree to a medication schedule that would allow her son to sleep pain-free for hours, with scheduled "alert time" so that he could confess and "be saved."

Many people find great comfort in the association of Christ's suffering with their own. Parents whose children are dying may find solace in thinking of God's suffering in the death of His son. Suffering in a Christian tradition that envisions the process of redemption and forgiveness may also impact human relationships. The following case illustrates this issue.

Lucy Guaterez is a 40-year-old homeless patient newly diagnosed with liver cancer. She reports that she has no living relatives. Her symptoms are controlled, but she is aware she likely will die in a matter of weeks. As the hospital social worker struggles to find a place for Lucy to live, given her multiple symptoms and complex medications, she finally confesses that her elderly mother lives nearby. They have not spoken in over 10 years; their relationship was destroyed because of Lucy's drug addictions. Lucy admitted to having stolen money from her mother and physically abusing her during the worst times of her life.

Lucy says she cannot call her mother but agrees to have the social worker make the call. Her mother, without hesitation, agrees to take in Lucy for the final weeks of her life. The hospice program assists in the transfer home and offers extra support, given the dynamics of the patient and her mother. Lucy does remarkably well once discharged to her mother's home, with the exception that her pain is not well-controlled. Her nausea and depression are much improved, and she enjoys her mother's cooking and sleeping in a soft bed. Until the last few days of life she tries to be independent, wanting to be as little burden as possible. The hospice has been able to meet Lucy's request for a daily home health aide visit for bathing. Lucy and her mother do not discuss the past and actually speak little. They spend considerable time sitting quietly together.

Frustrated by their inability to manage her pain, the hospice physician and nurses make numerous changes to her pain medications. In the weekly team meeting, the professional staff discuss the various drug options remaining. The home health aide interrupts to share her observation that although Lucy takes all of her own medications, she does rely on her mother to give pain medications. The aide further observes that Lucy only takes pain medicine if offered by her mother and then relies on her mother to decide if she should have one pill or two. One intense dynamic of this "prodigal daughter" seems clear: Lucy is asking for forgiveness from her mother in the form of pain medication.

Religious beliefs about suffering generally are based on scripture and family tradition and may be enacted in sacred ritual. For example, the Muslim tradition identifies suffering through the tradition of the Qur'an, recognizing God's divine power and the presence of illness or suffering as an aspect of life. The Qur'an and other sacred texts cite the story of Job and his appeal to God for relief from suffering. The Muslim faith values patience and devotion in times of suffering.

Faith traditions may teach about healing, miracles, and suffering. Death may be seen as a transition to a future existence. Islamic belief emphasizes the ultimate Will of God, whether it be in the form of surgery that extends life through a delicate procedure and highly advanced technology or in the form of supportive care if surgery is either unsuccessful or unwarranted.

One ICU nurse observed a Muslim family who waited patiently at the bedside of a teenage boy with acute renal failure from antibiotics given for a severe, untreated urinary tract infection. The family was just as diligent to regularly leave the ICU to pray in the adjacent waiting room. After a few days, the nurse felt comfortable enough with the family to comment about their devotion. She admitted she knew little about Islam, yet was quite moved by the family's persistent prayer for their son. The nurse was stunned to hear the father respond, "When we leave this room to pray, we are praying for you. We ask Muhammad to guide your hands on the dialysis machine so that you will save our son." The nurse first joked with her colleagues, "Imagine a Muslim praying for me, a Methodist!" Upon deeper reflection, the nurse shared how deeply touched she was by this Muslim prayer and how it caused her to reflect on her work not as a dialysis nurse "technician" but her role as a sacred healer and an instrument of God.

Another case illustrating the importance of culture follows.

An oncology nurse recalled a Chinese family who came to the patient's room every day with different herbal remedies, soups, and special foods to cure the patient's illness. The patient was a 35-year-old woman with recurring ovarian cancer. Upon discovery of the return of her cancer, her husband left her, knowing that she would not be able to provide him with the son he wanted. She had been admitted to the hospital previously for treatment; the chemotherapy, the surgery, and the days and nights spent in the hospital with uncontrolled symptoms were all familiar. Speaking very limited English, this patient always had a niece or nephew there to translate for her. Her family was very faithful. They went to the temple every weekend to pray for their beloved daughter, sister, aunt. They trusted that a higher power would help save her. They prayed at her bedside for her recovery. They believed that the bitterness of her life would be rewarded with health from this disease that they could not understand. It just simply could not be that "the one with white hair would send off the one with dark hair," that the daughter would die before the mother. Although the nurse did not know what the family's rituals meant or what kinds of foods they were feeding her, she understood that this ritual was necessary. It was their way of doing something. It was the only way they could accept what was happening before their eyes.

In the early 1900s, Max Scheler, a sociologist, wrote on the philosophy of religion and the concept of suffering. He described three major ways of dealing with suffering: *(1)* dulling it to the point of apathy, *(2)* struggling heroically against it, and *(3)* suppressing it to the point of believing it is an illusion. He contrasts Christian perspectives of suffering as redemptive and Christ-like with the Buddhist views of suffering as an opportunity for understanding and insight (Bershady, 1992). Scheler's work is a reminder of the importance of cultural consideration and assessing individual responses to common medical diagnosis.

There are extensive resources to guide nurses in understanding various religious perspectives on illness and death and on specific issues such as organ transplantation, autopsy, care of the body after death, and grieving (Berry and Griffe, 2006; Puchalski et al., 2004; Kagawa-Singer, 1994). Beyond the specific details of each religion or tradition lies the important common need for nurses to respect diverse cultures and to support patients and families in their faith traditions.

Each of the stories in this chapter illustrates the importance of relationship. Nurses offer relief of suffering through presence. They offer compassion and trust. There are few real "quick fixes" in nursing. Nonetheless, nurses are performing sacred work as they remain steadfast in the face of impossible suffering. They help to find meaning in that suffering, seek and grant forgiveness, and transcend even the worst of life circumstances. As Weatherhead said:

> The man who inquires into the problem of suffering may be compared with one who from some sunny street, steps into the comparative gloom of a vast cathedral. After the blaze outside, all seems dark. As his eyes grow accustomed to the darkness he notices unsuspected windows which throw light upon the way he treads . . . and in the end there is no darkness to make him afraid. (Weatherhead, 1936, 25)

SACRED ACTS IN THE ABSENCE OF RELIGION

Marvin Wilson is a 62-year-old African-American man who went through a bitter divorce 3 years ago. Marvin and his ex-wife Gail have not been on speaking terms since their separation. Both fought bitterly in dividing their property, and their two adult daughters became enemies as they each took sides with one of the parents. These past years have included hostile interactions, court appearances, restraining orders, and police visits. Both Marvin and Gail have since remarried. Marvin just weeks ago sustained a critical spine injury after diving into a shallow pool. He is now quadriplegic and has a brain-stem injury. He is comatose and ventilator-dependent. After extensive deliberation and consultation, a decision is made to discontinue his life support and allow him to die.

In the first week of his hospitalization, the daughters argued angrily, and hospital security was called on at least three occasions. Since then, as the reality of their father's prognosis has sunken in and exhaustion has replaced hostility, the family members have remained separated but become more peaceful. The families decline any chaplaincy involvement. Marvin had no prior religious affiliation and, when interviewed, Marvin's new wife said she "used to believe in God" but that "there is no God if a man as good as Marvin is allowed to die."

All of the extended family members and the daughters and their respective spouses ask to be present as Marvin's life support is discontinued. A joint decision is made about a funeral home, but the nurse is aware that the families are planning separate funeral services.

Recognizing the impact and power of stopping the ventilator and Marvin's subsequent death, the nurse is also aware of the absence of any ritual, prayer, or other sacred acts. On this, the entire family seems to agree. After he dies, the nurse notices that the daughters linger behind. She asks if they would like to stay and help her bathe and dress Marvin before the mortuary comes. In absolute silence but constant tears, each daughter takes a side of his body, guided gently by the instruction of the nurse as their father's body is cleaned and prepared.

Even in the absence of religion, faith community, or a recognized ritual, nurses have the ability to bring a sense of humanity even in the most difficult of circumstances. Nurses are guided by ethical perspectives that extend beyond professional codes and call upon basic human kindness and compassion as they are called to embrace spirituality in its most global sense. Nurses hear confessions, perform "baptisms," affirm faith, and support the process of forgiveness, all within the context of their daily work.

The expert nurse knows that much redemption happens when a hostile family member assists in a bath. Nurses know that asking the frightened husband to spoon-feed his spouse a few sips of soup or coaching a grandson to massage the back of his grandfather are more than physical acts. They are sacred acts and they are actions that become the life-long memories of those who live beyond the illness or death of a loved one.

SUMMARY

The understanding of suffering from a nursing perspective has been enriched by the work of scholars in the fields of ethics and theology. An early nursing contribution to the exploration of suffering included research conducted by Battenfield (1984), who used qualitative methods to develop an operational schema of suffering through interviews of nine patients facing serious illness. She concluded her paper by saying:

> Nurses, long accepted as comforters in time of human need, have developed and refined multiple skills, arts, and knowledge to enable them to alleviate suffering at times of physical pain and emotional upheaval. Perhaps the suffering schema, as a small addendum to their bag of tools and rules, could lend an enriched awareness to the concept of suffering and expand the nurse's ability to aid fellow human beings to climb from a depth of turmoil to the height of a mind at peace. (Battenfield, 1984, 40)

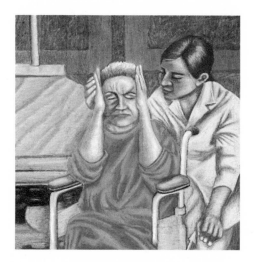

CHAPTER 3 ❧

Contextual Analysis of Patient Suffering

An examination of suffering as an intensely personal, whole-person experience can best be done, in part, through narratives of suffering individuals. In this chapter, we attempt a contextual analysis of suffering through narratives written by nurses, patients, and their families. Other sources include professional literature and our prior research conducted at the City of Hope National Medical Center.

Before exploring specific patient contexts, a useful framework through which to consider suffering is a QOL model (Ferrell, 1996). QOL encompasses four dimensions of well-being: physical, psychological, social, and spiritual (Figure 3.1). In some ways, the dimensions are relatively distinct; however, there is also tremendous overlap. Physical symptoms such as pain clearly have an impact on psychological symptoms such as anxiety. Physical and psychological distress may also affect spiritual well-being. A patient with increasing pain may be reminded of the imminence of death. Pain may then become a message of transcendence. Patients with renal failure who unexpectedly receive successful kidney transplants see their physical symptoms resolve, yet they may also feel guilty for having survived when so many others do not. The question "Why me?" applies just as commonly for those succumbing to life-threatening illness as for those who have survived such an illness. Each individual's answer to that question may have a powerful impact on the other dimensions of well-being.

The contexts of suffering included here are: Pain, Oncology, Critical Care, Pediatrics, Geriatrics, and Family Caregivers. These contexts are then

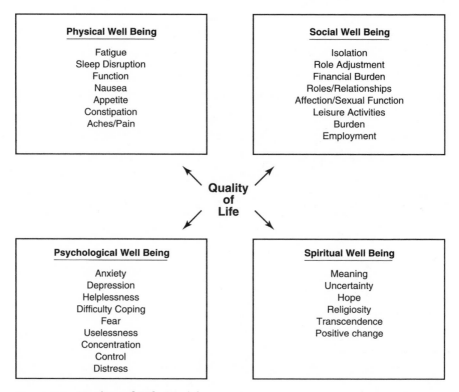

Figure 3.1. Quality of Life Model

explored both in terms of common themes and in terms of the goals of nursing in caring for individuals under these circumstances.

THE CONTEXT OF PAIN

The presence of pain is almost never an isolated symptom but is a whole-person experience. People in pain may move from a usual state of health—in which the body is largely ignored—to a state of constant and distressing awareness of physical sensations. Steeves (1988) conducted research in the early years of bone marrow transplantation used to treat hematologic malignancies. He documented suffering associated with common transplant toxicities, including mucositis, pain from multiple causes, and other symptoms. He found that patients sometimes coped with extreme pain through the phenomenon of "downward social compassion," which involved coping through thinking of others whose plight was worse than their own. They also coped through a sense of altruism, believing their suffering would benefit science and would greatly diminish the suffering of future patients.

They relied extensively on religion, sometimes equating their experiences to Job, who appealed to God to make meaning of his suffering. Job's suffering was recognized by these patients as severe and seemed without purpose, similar to their own experiences (Steeves, 1988).

The phrase "pain and suffering" is so commonly used that we often think of these two phenomena—*pain* and *suffering*—as one (Baines and Norlander, 2000; Chapman and Gavrin, 1999; Hill, 1992). This is interesting because medical care has so often been criticized for separating the mind and body (Cassell, 1991). Although pain and suffering are separate experiences that can certainly exist in the absence of the other, understanding suffering in the context of pain is useful.

Cassell's paper on suffering and the goals of medicine emphasizes the topic of pain. Cassell says that suffering occurs when people in pain feel out of control, when the pain is overwhelming, when the source of pain is unknown, when the meaning of pain is dire, or when the pain is chronic (Cassell, 1982, 641). Pain may be perceived as a threat to continued existence and to the person's integrity as a whole being. In this article on "The Nature of Suffering and the Goals of Medicine," the recommendations for relieving suffering, even in the presence of continued pain, are most profound. Here, Cassell says that the necessary elements are " . . . making the source of pain known, changing its meaning, demonstrating that it can be controlled, and that an end is in sight" (Cassell, 1982, 641). Nurses are called on every day to offer these very elements of comfort. These are common activities for nurses.

Nurses are a voice for patients in pain. Dr. Laurel Archer Copp wrote "Treatment, Torture, Suffering and Compassion," challenging nurses to prevent pain whenever possible, to respond aggressively when pain occurs, and to be compassionate when pain persists (Copp, 1990b). Nurses have been advocates for improved pain management and have been among the first to address ethical perspectives of our failure to relieve pain. In 1990, Meinhart and McCaffery wrote that " . . . failure to treat pain is inhumane and constitutes professional negligence." A few years later, in 1994, the first national guidelines for pain management were released (Agency for Health Care Policy and Research, 1994), calling on professionals to address the serious issue of undertreated pain.

Pain associated with cancer and terminal illness has been extensively addressed (Loeser, 2000). The severity of cancer's physical pain often leads to thoughts of death. As the patient begins to recognize the multitude of losses that death brings, physical pain may be experienced more as suffering. In a grounded theory study of pain in elderly patients with cancer, Duggleby concluded that suffering is the basic social problem of pain and that the patients she interviewed dealt with pain through "enduring." Trusting in a higher being and finding meaning in the pain were ways of maintaining the hope necessary to endure (Duggleby, 2000).

Nurses understand pain far beyond tissue injury, diseased organs, or neurophysiology, and they have described human experiences of pain (Stark and McGovern, 1992; Rodgers and Cowles, 1997; Spross, 1996). Table 3.1 depicts a selection of these narratives. Nurses require expert skills in communication as they respond to patients who are suffering with the common perception that pain is God's Will (Kumasaka and Miles, 1996).

Table 3.1. A Selection of Narratives of Patients in Pain As Shared by Nurses

The patient was an 83-year-old lady with metastatic breast and ovarian cancer. She spoke of continual pain although there seemed to be no identifiable reason for pain. In a series of three conversations, this patient began to express a history of spousal sexual assault resulting in pregnancy. This pregnancy was then terminated by her husband in their home. She had never spoken of this and had never dealt with her feeling of shame and her feelings of grief for her unborn child. We spoke at length and planned a service for her child. Three hours following a very private service this patient's symptoms were eased. Her anxiety had dissipated and her death was peaceful. Her suffering was eased!

A 32-year-old male diagnosed with advanced AIDS was in an "isolation" room. The male was presently alert and oriented. His body was frail and very emaciated. His lips were swollen and his mouth had multiple sores. His sacral area had stage 3–4 decubitus, the anal area was bright red and seeping with liquid BM. He was beginning to have contractures and open decubiti were on both heels. The gastronomy tube was in place. The site was raw. The foley catheter was barely draining. The nausea was persistent. He was in obvious pain, but brave.

I had a patient with end-stage pancreatic cancer. He begged me to control his pain, stating he didn't care if he died. "Just stop the pain." Eventually, he died in pain. I had visited this patient 6 days/week for 3 weeks. He had faith in me. We both suffered when I couldn't improve his pain. I was hurting for him. He could barely speak, because he was in so much pain.

He was recently released from prison on a compassionate release with weeks to live, diagnosed with lung cancer. He was homeless, but had a one-week voucher for a shelter. He was admitted to inpatient hospice for severe right shoulder pain. His suffering was from being inside, not in his familiar environment (the streets by day, the canyon at night) and feeling he was still "incarcerated" and not in control of his life. This was a surprise. We thought his suffering would be from his past misdeeds, failures in life, estrangement from family. But he suffered because he was inside, although technically "free!"

A father and husband in his 40s had much difficulty getting his pain under control. He had always been active and very involved and was no longer able to fill the role he had been in for so long.

A patient said, "The pain is terrible, why don't you just kill me?"

The patient told us, "The pain was so bad yesterday, if I had a gun I would have shot myself. It's better now."

The problem of untreated pain was explored using a framework of feminist ethics (Ferrell, 2005). While the field of feminist ethics applies to all aspects and concepts of suffering, it is particularly relevant to pain when recognizing its key concepts such as nurturance, compassion, and communication (Welch, 2000). Feminist ethics has articulated the need to address patterns of oppression, domination, and violence (Tong, 1993), words that also describe the experience of pain and associated suffering. Those professionals who hold the ability to relieve pain through prescribing or administering medications are clearly in a dominant position over the vulnerable person awaiting relief from pain. The failure to relieve pain and the infliction of pain have been cited as forms of violence.

Understanding patient experiences as physiological processes (pain) as well as human phenomenon (suffering) is an essential aspect of a nurse's responsibility to relieve pain. Applying the feminist concept of relationship, we can recognize the intimacy of the patient–nurse relationship as analgesic. The concept of relationship includes the intimate personal connections between individuals. In *The Body in Pain*, Elaine Scarry (1985) eloquently described the vulnerability of the human as a body in pain. Such a human is often dominated and oppressed by the health-care system. The patient may be silent and without ability to express the emotions (suffering) of pain. Scarry is most often quoted for her "model of certainty," which describes those in pain as being very certain of the presence and impact of the pain, and her "model of doubt," which describes the caregivers who often underestimate or deny the pain of another (Scarry, 1985).

Pain that is diminished, ignored, or doubted is pain that leads to suffering. Nurses, therefore, have a moral imperative to advocate for pain relief, give voice to pain, and reduce suffering (Greipp, 1992; Ersek and Ferrell, 1994). This may be complicated by power dynamics in relationships, as feminist ethicists have described (Held, 1995), which frequently occur when the vulnerable depend on dominant forces within systems of injustice. Even the most compassionate nurse has social dominance over vulnerable patients in pain, the power to accept or doubt the pain, and access to pain medications that could provide relief. There is strong evidence that vulnerable populations such as children, the poor, elderly, women, those who do not speak English, and anyone with a history of substance abuse are much more likely to get inadequate treatment of pain (Agency for Health Care Policy and Research, 1994).

Considering the power dynamics that exist in patient–provider relationships, it is also important to acknowledge that the nurse can also be the one who inflicts pain. One of the few researchers to investigate the phenomenon of inflicted pain is Irene Madjar, who at the time of the study was a doctoral student in Canada. The study "Giving Comfort and Inflicting

Pain" thoughtfully explored pain caused by nurses (Madjar, 1998). Her study included patients suffering from burns and those with cancer who were undergoing chemotherapy. Madjar noted that patients experienced painful procedures as "wounding" and medical instruments as "weapons." Patients believed that nurses varied tremendously in their basic approach to caring for patients' bodies. The touch of a nurse was described as engendering trust and comfort, or conversely, the nurse's touch could cause tension and distress, thus directly influencing the physical and psychological experience of the patient. This was particularly true for the patients with burns in Madjar's study.

Madjar found that the touch of nurses during "inflicted pain" had significant impact on patients, and they defined qualities of the "good nurses" as gentleness, trustworthiness, sensitivity, technical competence, knowledge, and skillful communication. A nurse with these qualities made patients feel special, cared for, encouraged, and reassured. Madjar concluded that "wanting to care and having to inflict pain are dissonant and not easily reconcilable facets of nurses' work with patients in acute hospital settings" (Madjar, 1998, 159). She asserted that without systematic support, nurses were left to resolve this dissonance for themselves.

The concept of compassion also deserves discussion for its relevance to nursing care of patients in pain. Feminist scholar Margaret Farley (2002) described true compassion as a "spiritual act" and stated that compassion is to go with the person in pain and stay there with the suffering person. Theologian Henri Nouwen (1991) similarly wrote of compassion and the concept of suffering with the other. Managing pain is far more than the giving of pain medication. Nurses demonstrate compassion as they listen to the patient's description of pain, validate its presence and importance, and offer their commitment to relieving the pain. The varied approaches of different nurses to a patient in pain undoubtedly impact that patient's perception and experience of pain.

Nurses have led efforts within institutions, professional nursing organizations, and interdisciplinary programs to improve pain relief. These efforts have addressed acute and postoperative pain, chronic pain, and pain from life-threatening diseases. Making improvements in pain policy and in clinical practice has often required almost militant action, beginning with strong voices to overcome "models of doubt," as described by Scarry (1985), and insisting on aggressive measures to relieve pain, particularly in vulnerable populations. Welch, a professor of Women's Studies and Religious Studies, has described "courageous acts of resistance," in which agents of change defeat injustice and domination (Welch, 2000). Her concept of "communities of resistance" applies to nurses who individually and collectively have advocated for pain relief.

Jewish literature has also contributed to our understanding of suffering, often through narratives of experiences in the Holocaust. Raphael, a scholar in theology, wrote a profound book titled *The Female Face of God in Auschwitz* (2003), offering a feminist perspective of the Holocaust. Raphael addresses the common notion that God is absent in horrific conditions such as those of Auschwitz. She describes women who care for the sick and dying in the concentration camps as *"the face of God."* She writes of the compassionate touch of women as they comforted their physically devastated companion prisoners as they died.

Over the last 40 years, the most prominent voice advocating for improved pain management has been a nurse, Margo McCaffery. Until McCaffery wrote of pain (McCaffery, 1968) and began what has been nearly 40 years of writing and lecturing on the topic, pain was defined in physiologic terms and with an emphasis on the dominant role of professionals to determine if a patient was in pain. McCaffery's redefinition of pain was both simple and profound. Her internationally recognized definition that "pain is what the person says it is, existing whenever he or she says it does" has been a voice for the feminist principle of respect (Cannon, 1995; Jaggar, 1989).

The politics of power and domination in health care have resulted in a system in which women and others have been systematically undertreated for pain. In a brilliant analysis of this subject titled "The Girl Who Cried Pain: A Bias Against Women in the Treatment of Pain," authors Hoffman and Tarzian (2001) analyze historical contexts, social structures, and biological literature to document the undertreatment of women's pain. The authors cite a Christian context of pain as found in Genesis 3:16, "To the woman, God said, 'I will greatly multiply your pain in child bearing; in pain you shall bring forth children, yet your desire shall be for your husband, and he shall rule over you.'"

Feminist scholar Katie Cannon (1995) describes the African-American woman's experience when she discusses the physical abuse of slaves. Cannon articulates the need to overcome the force of domination and ". . . deliverance from the discursive silence that society at large has used to deny the basis of shared humanity." Feminist scholar and philosopher Alison Jaggar (1989) has used the term "outlaw emotions" to describe the problem of alienation when, for example, women in pain cannot express their suffering for fear of alienating themselves from professionals on whom they depend.

The essence of feminist ethics applied to the problem of pain is captured in writing by Farley (2002). In her thoughtful text, *Compassionate Respect: A Feminist Approach to Medical Ethics and Other Questions*, Farley argues that our current ethical approaches are built solely on the principle

of autonomy, shifting the burden to the patient and disregarding professional obligations for compassionate action. She wrote of "compassionate
respect," which should be a moral response to ameliorate suffering or—
at the very least—to witness it with that same compassion. She acknowledges great disparities in current contexts of care, such as those living with
HIV/AIDS. She concludes that feminist ethics requires care to be "respectful of embodied autonomy as well as every level of need in the person
to whom care is owed" (Farley, 2002, 43).

The lessons of feminist scholarship apply equally to care of men in pain.
While the vulnerable groups described earlier are often undertreated, one
can argue that all people in pain are vulnerable. Living in untreated pain
diminishes the person, immobilizes both physical and cognitive function,
and causes the suffering person to question the value of life and their faith
beliefs. Every inadequate or denied dose of pain medication is a reminder
that the very human experience of a body certain of its pain, as described by
Scarry (1985), has been ignored. Pain potentiates more pain, and unrelieved
pain diminishes the human to profound depths of emotional and physical
dependence.

Our ability to relieve pain should be the litmus test of our value as
health-care professionals. It is the core of our contract with society and the
mandate of our privilege to be nurses. The profession of nursing could
benefit from greater emphasis on the relief of pain as a fundamental human
right.

THE CONTEXT OF CANCER

Analogous to the association of "pain and suffering" is the association of
"cancer and death." Despite advances in earlier detection, treatment, and
cancer survivorship, hearing the words "You have cancer" is almost always
heard as a death sentence. The prevalence and visibility of cancer are two
social factors in the fear of a cancer diagnosis. Virtually everyone knows
someone with cancer and has witnessed the devastating effects of the disease. Most people also know of someone who has died from cancer. Unfortunately, the collective memory of society often is of people they have
known who died in pain.

Another major factor in the association of cancer and suffering is the
recognition of the caustic effects of cancer treatments. There is well-
deserved recognition that even with the best prognosis, the effects of surgery, chemotherapy, or radiation therapy are distressing and can be devastating. There is a legacy of cancer in which many people diagnosed with
cancer are soon reminded of the public images of those who have died from

the disease or of personal experiences of witnessing cancer's effects and the effects of treatment on a loved one. In our research related to women with ovarian cancer, an unfortunately large number of these women shared stories of witnessing their own mothers or grandmothers die from ovarian cancer and in agonizing pain. There is an enormous need for health-care professionals to reverse this legacy so that future patients will have legacies of compassionate care and comfort.

SUFFERING IN CANCER SURVIVORSHIP

The suffering associated with cancer is examined first in the context of those living with or "surviving" cancer and is followed by a discussion of advanced cancer and living in the shadow of death. All phases of cancer across the trajectory of diagnosis, treatment, remission, or recurrence are associated with suffering.

There is often a perception that suffering is limited to advanced cancer or to the final months of life as the physical body declines and the living person becomes a dying person. The Institute of Medicine's 2005 report, "From Cancer Patient to Cancer Survivor: Lost in Transition," recognizes that there are now over 10 million cancer survivors in the United States. The suffering of these individuals across the trajectory from initial diagnosis, treatment, remission, and even long-term survival is enormous. Cancer, at even the earliest stage, with the best treatment, leading to the best response and most optimistic prognosis is . . . cancer (Charmaz, 1983). We, as health-care providers, often believe that if our care is good, suffering can be avoided. While suffering can be heard, validated, and diminished, it remains a common response to serious illness and death.

On surviving cancer, Mullan says:

> Despite this success on the treatment front, we have done very little in a concerted and well-planned fashion to investigate and address the problems of survivors. It is as if we have invented sophisticated techniques to save people from drowning, but once they have been pulled from the water, we leave them on the dock to cough and splutter on their own in the belief that we have done all we can. (Mullan, 1985, 273)

Researchers and psychosocial clinicians have explored the phenomenon of cancer survivorship. Their work has consistently revealed that cancer survivors report not only physical effects of the disease such as lingering fatigue but also the effects of living with an altered body after surgery or reconstructing a life after the traumatic diagnosis of cancer. They also share the existential crisis of a cancer diagnosis and the search to make meaning from their illness and loss and how to live well with an uncertain future. The effects on family members of patients with cancer are equally distressing (Northouse et al., 2002; Lewis and Deal, 1995; Morse and Fife, 1998).

There is growing awareness that cancer survivorship is also a time of deep spiritual meaning. Surviving cancer may mean becoming closer to God or one's faith to "get through" the treatment. Faith can offer a protection against the enduring threat that cancer will return.

Alan is a 30-year-old Jewish man. He had a slight head injury during a tennis game and is seen in the ER. An X-ray reveals a mass in his brain that is believed to be a brain tumor.

Alan says that although he has been raised in a very devout Jewish family grounded in multiple generations of religious life, his own faith diminished in early adulthood and his only affiliations at the Temple are social in nature, void of any deep meaning. Having had what he described as a "dress rehearsal" for death, Alan becomes deeply involved in his faith and as an active leader in the Temple. As he returns to an active spiritual life, he encounters many others in his religious community who share a recent life-altering experience that led to their return to formal involvement in their faith. Participating in Rosh Hashanah for the first time after his illness touches him more profoundly than he ever would have imagined.

Alan says a nursing assistant in the hospital radiology department was his "Rabbi." The nursing assistant, Ben, is also Jewish and met Alan on his initial ER visit when his mass was discovered. The men share humorous stories of growing up Jewish, which Alan finds to be of great benefit as a distraction amidst the anxiety producing tests. In the weeks that follow, as Alan returns for more diagnostic tests, their conversations become more serious. Alan confides his growing remorse about having abandoned his family heritage. Ben becomes his "Rabbi" as Alan "practices" on Ben what he plans to say to the Temple Rabbi about his return to the faith community. Ben "mostly listens" as Alan talks but also offers to pray for Alan.

After an additional 3 weeks, which he describes as "torturous," Alan is told that the mass is benign and that he requires no further treatment. When Alan receives the biopsy report confirming the unexpected good news, he makes a trip back to the hospital just to thank Ben for his support. Still overwhelmed by the news, Alan says he needs another week to absorb it all, to get his emotions in check before going to his Temple. He gives Ben a donation to his Temple and asks if he could pass it on as an offering of thanks.

This case illustrates one of the many opportunities for health-care professionals to be present to people amidst life crisis as they face their own mortality and revisit their faith traditions. In this case, Ben's genuine compassion and sharing of mutual faith experiences was a vital force in Alan's weeks of suffering and now in his re-evalutation of life priorities.

Juarez and colleagues studied perceptions of QOL in Hispanic patients with cancer and concluded that belief in God was an essential aspect of spirituality (Juarez, Ferrell, and Borneman, 1998). In the words of two of the Hispanic cancer survivors:

> I take it with a lot of peace, my illness. If that's what I deserve, so be it. I tell Him, 'Wait a little while, at least give me a few days to feel good, and then, You must know if you are going to call me, You know what you are doing.'

> I have to endure this illness, I welcome it. Why? Because that's God's law. I have put myself in God's hands. The day He knocks on my door and tells me, 'Now,' here I am.

Survivorship is often a time of optimistic living complicated by the fear of recurrence. There is deep angst in confronting the reality of all that has happened since cancer was diagnosed, feeling the emotions of surviving life-threatening treatments and now reclaiming life as a survivor. Even with the most optimistic of prognoses after cancer treatment, cancer survivors know life is forever changed.

In addition to the existential crisis of cancer survivorship, there is extensive support for the notion that having cancer and surviving cancer often strengthen faith and improve QOL. When the physical body is devastated, social supports are tested, and there are overwhelming psychological effects of disease and treatment. Spiritual well-being becomes a control aspect of survivorship (Ferrell, Grant, Funk, Otis-Green, and Garcia, 1997; Ferrell, Dow, Leigh, Ly, and Gulasekaram, 1995).

In a synthesis of literature related to the meaning of survivorship, several themes are relevant for understanding suffering in this context. Survivors seek a sense of wholeness after what is almost uniformly described as a life-altering experience. Achieving wholeness includes creating a sense of life purpose with the identity as a "cancer survivor" and begs the questions "Who am I? What is the purpose of my life? Why did I survive?" (Dow, Ferrell, Haberman, and Eaton, 1999).

Surviving cancer causes many people to believe that *quality of life* simply means having a life—just being alive. Survivors struggle to place the cancer within the context of their life rather than having cancer consume their lives. The fact of having survived is met by a profound search for meaning (Dow et al., 1999). Suffering also occurs in cancer survivorship as a result of loss of finances, relationships, function, sexuality, and fertility. Another theme of cancer survivorship described was that "quality of life in survivorship means gaining a sense of control in life rather than being controlled by cancer" (Dow et al., 1999).

In recent years, Lance Armstrong (Tour de France world champion cyclist) has become the public image of cancer survivorship. The image of survivorship often implies a state of normalcy, a return to health, and that cancer is "over." This public image is ironic in that Lance Armstrong himself, and the foundation in his name, is devoted to awareness and advocacy of the unique needs of cancer survivors. Lance Armstrong and his foundation are recognized not only for advocating early detection and cure but also for being a moral voice in honestly addressing what many cancer organizations have attempted to deny: people living beyond cancer have enormous physical, psychosocial, and spiritual needs, and even when cancer is cured, it isn't "over." Cancer alters the meaning of life forever.

Surviving cancer with an excellent prognosis, such as early stage breast or prostate cancer, is challenging, but surviving a cancer with likely recurrence and poor long-term survival can create enormous suffering (Arman et al., 2002; Ferrell, Smith, Juarez, and Melancon, 2003). Women with ovarian cancer clearly illustrate this situation. As a result of treatment advances, more than 200,000 women now live with ovarian cancer. These women are profoundly aware that the likelihood of recurrence is high. People living with other progressive chronic illness for whom death may not be imminent but is nonetheless a feared aspect of the disease may find themselves in circumstances similar to cancer survivors (Ganzini, Johnston, and Hoffman, 1999).

Suffering from ovarian cancer begins with the recognition that this cancer is typically diagnosed late in the course of disease, with more than 75% of women already at advanced stages of the cancer from the time of diagnosis. This fact alone compounds suffering in many ways. Although ovarian cancer has been described as a "silent disease," many ovarian cancer survivors have spoken strongly to say that it isn't the disease that is silent; rather, the medical system simply hasn't been listening (Ersek, Ferrell, Dow, and Melancon, 1997).

In an analysis of over 21,000 letters written by ovarian cancer survivors to a newsletter support group (Ferrell, Smith, Juarez, and Melancon, 2003), essential views of the suffering of women with ovarian cancer have been identified (Table 3.2). This table summarizes key themes from these letters,

Table 3.2. The Meaning of Illness and Spirituality in Ovarian Cancer Survivors

Religious Practices and Experiences

AAA could not be called to route a new course. A repairman could not be sent out to replace a worn out part. Only God could give me what I needed . . . strength, hope, courage, peace, and joy in the midst of the storm.

I believe there are no coincidences, only God-incidences. My blessings are too many to count. I have so much love in my heart, my cup runneth over. I have enough love for many who are newly diagnosed or just plain afraid no matter how long they have been fighting this war, for I have walked in their shoes. I just keep putting one foot in front of the other. I am never alone, for as so many of us have found, "We can't give it away, for we receive so much more than we give."

My doctors are amazed I'm holding on. One asked me what church I go to. He said he would love to join. They scratch their heads and wonder. I do have faith, and God is my physician.

I look at my cancer as a test from God. That's okay, I just would like to know what the question was!

As Christmas approached, my husband and I talked about what I wanted for Christmas. I felt I wanted something that would remind me each day of all my blessings and give me strength to make it through the next six months. We came up with the idea of a blessing bracelet with four charms: a cross to remind me of my faith and that God was walking with me, a heart to remind me of my love for God and my family and friends and their love for me, an angel to remind me that I had a guardian angel and that I was never alone, and a dove to remind me that peace would be mine if I would remember what the symbols meant.

Spiritual Activities and Experiences

Follow inner guidance. The Western medical folks are good at surgery. But other treatments are harsh and based on statistics. No one is a statistic. Everybody and every life is individual. It is the inner guidance that is essential for tailoring actions to what each person needs and what the soul desires.

I meditated; joined a cancer group; talked to other women battling cancer all over the country and globe; prayed; forgave and asked forgiveness from all those I'd wronged either real or imagined; stayed pretty connected to my family and close and good friends; avoided or limited contact with negative souls and thoughts; visualized a healing taking place; listened to inspirational tapes, emotionally satisfying music; sought out beauty everywhere; gave thanks for all my blessings; and acknowledged knowing that I was healed through faith even before it was medically confirmed when my gynecologic oncologist/surgeon could not find any cancer during my "second look" surgery. Today, I still give thanks daily for my healing both spiritually and physically. I stay in contact with those near and dear to me. I work out of my home with its soothing, healing, breathtaking view of the Pacific Ocean to remind me that we all are spiritual beings who have chosen a physical experience here and now, and "in this moment" I am well and I am happy.

Negative Changes in Spirituality

I was mad at God! I said this is not fair. Why am I going through this? I hadn't even had a good life—no grandchildren—why! Why! I am going to be very mad when I get to heaven.

(continued)

Table 3.2. *(continued)*

But where do we go from here? Do we just sit by and let that insidious ovarian cancer creep through our abdomens in thin sheets, covering all our organs and choking out our lives?

I'm having a hard time accepting this and at times do pray I die.

Positive Changes in Spirituality

For my life now, I am definitely a happier person than I was prediagnosis. I have a greater appreciation for all of the pleasures, big and small, that living has to offer. For about the past 15 years, I had stopped celebrating my birthday. I hated growing older, felt that the best years were behind me, and was not particularly looking forward to 50 and beyond. As I mentioned, I celebrated my 48th birthday in the hospital. All of a sudden I confronted the alternative to not celebrating another year of life—and believe me, I know which is a better choice! Last year's birthday celebration began at midnight and lasted for days. This year I intend to give great thanks for having the opportunity to celebrate turning 50!

However, I am determined not to sit down or lie down and let this thing get me. I am going to *live* until I die—however long that is.

Emotionally, I am also much better. I now take joy in such small things—a beautiful snowfall, cottony clouds in the sky, the ability to walk quickly up a flight of stairs without becoming completely exhausted when I reach the top.

Purpose in Survivorship

There is nothing like a purpose, a calling, a mission, a goal, a cause, or a self-chosen desire to help others to give us survival power.

Hopefulness

Cancer is like a traffic jam on a hot August day. You want to get on with your life, but you creep inch by inch, feeling trapped and all alone. Waiting for whatever it is that is blocking you from the rest of your life to disappear. Yelling and screaming does not make the traffic go away. You become discouraged, anxious, and tired. Then, just when you think you will be in that jam forever, the roadblock clears, the traffic begins to move a little faster, and you start to feel a sense of hope. You realize that you will eventually get to where you are going, a little slower than you had anticipated and maybe on a different road, but you will get there. It's a long and lonely trip to make by yourself.

Adapted with permission from Ferrell, B. R., S. L. Smith, G. Juarez, and C. Melancon. (2003). Meaning of illness and spirituality in ovarian cancer survivors. *Oncology Nursing Forum.* 30: 249–257.

including findings that confronting this disease creates both positive and negative responses.

The now-prominent cancer survivorship movement with 10 million constituents emerged as a quiet voice only 20 years ago. Dr. Mullan, a physician diagnosed with cancer, chronicled his experiences in what has become a classic paper published in the *New England Journal of Medicine* titled, "Seasons of Survival: Reflections of a Physician with Cancer." Mullan wrote:

> As with most cancer patients, the quality of my life during this period was severely compromised, and the possibility of death was always present. I was, in fact, surviving, struggling physically and mentally with the cancer, the therapy, and the large scale disruption in my life. Survival, however, was not one condition but many. It was desperate days of nausea and depression. It was elation at the birth of a daughter in the midst of treatment. It was the anxiety of waiting for my monthly chest film to be taken and lying awake nights feeling for lymph nodes. It was the joy of eating Chinese food for the first time after battling radiation burns of the esophagus for four months. These reflections and many others are a jumble of memories of a purgatory that was touched by sickness in all its aspects but was neither death nor cure. It was survival—an absolutely predictable but ill-defined condition that all cancer patients pass through as they struggle with their illness. (Mullan, 1985, 271)

Surviving cancer, similarly to surviving other catastrophic events or traumatic circumstances in life, leaves an indelible mark on the soul of the person who has suffered.

The guilty feelings of Holocaust survivors mirror the guilt of the woman who has survived breast cancer when she attends a breast cancer survivor's meeting only to learn of the loss of a fellow patient. Surviving cancer means asking not only "Why did I get cancer?" but also "Why did I survive?" This statement has been spoken by many who have survived bone marrow transplants, particularly in the earliest years of the treatment, when mortality was high (Grant, et al., 1992).

The many emotions of cancer survivorships are illustrated in the words of a long-term breast cancer survivor, written more than a decade after her diagnosis. She shared:

> The "why" questions are a whole subject into themselves. In my experience, faith helps one to realize that "why" questions are not useful because they don't have answers. In fact, the "why" of this disease and its cure is mysterious. Faith helps me to live with the mystery, to move out of "why?" to a (for me) more useful question: "where is God in this experience?" Also, in truth, asking "why me?" is like asking about any lottery win. The answer is: "why not me?" To acknowledge our vulnerability to the biological hand of the universe is very scary!

SUFFERING IN ADVANCED CANCER

Advanced cancer has served as a model for studying the concept of suffering. With more than 570,000 cancer deaths each year in the United States (American Cancer Society, 2006), suffering in advanced cancer is all too common. Advances in the provision of cancer care, which offer excellent physical care and symptom management combined with psychological, social, and spiritual care, have allowed for the ability to minimize suffering to the greatest extent possible.

There is remarkable consistency in studies describing the experience of suffering in advanced cancer (Cherny, Coyle, and Foley, 1994; Chochinov, Hack, and Hussard, 2002). Researchers in diverse settings have interviewed patients with cancer and consistently concluded that suffering exists across dimensions of physical, psychological/emotional, social/interpersonal, and spiritual/existential well-being (Benedict, 1989; Kuuppelomaki and Sirkka, 1998; Battenfield, 1984; O'Connor, Wicker, and Germino, 1990). The physical devastation of cancer, the presence of pain and other symptoms, and the caustic impact of treatments often lead to social isolation, which results in further withdrawal and isolation.

Coyle (1996) described emotional responses of patients with advanced cancer through a synthesis of interviews and research with patients suffering from cancer. Table 3.3 includes powerful images through the voices of people with advanced cancer.

Coyle recently published a paper titled "The Hard Work of Living in the Face of Death" (2006). This phenomenological study captures the essence of simultaneously living with advanced cancer and facing the immediacy of death. Coyle describes the hard work of tasks such as maintaining control, creating a system of support and safety, finding meaning, and creating a legacy (Coyle, 2006).

Nurses play an essential role throughout the disease process in reducing the suffering of cancer. Recognizing losses and speaking of them ranges from circumstances such as our patient's loss of hair in initial chemotherapy to the loss of role when the patient becomes too weak to hold a grandchild. Suffering is acknowledged and sometimes reduced by the act of comforting as we give voice and a listening presence to the suffering.

There is tremendous variation in the needs of dying patients, and even as death approaches, patients are people—people who are incredibly individual in how they die:

One of my (Ferrell) first patients as a hospice volunteer was a 90-year-old woman dying of pancreatic cancer. She had become progressively weak and was confined to bed but had been instructed to do simple exercises in

and highly skilled in guiding patients and families through the psychological and spiritual crisis of life-threatening acute illness and injury. Dr. Bernice Harper has devoted a career to studying the stages of adaptation by expert nurses working with serious illness (Harper, 1994). She has defined six stages of adaptation: intellectualization, emotional survival, depression, emotional arrival, deep compassion, and the final stage, labeled the "do-er," in which the nurse is able to care for patients and families while also caring for him- or herself. Nurses in critical-care settings require spiritual reflection and replenishment to sustain their expert care (Davies, 2006).

PEDIATRICS: THE SUFFERING OF CHILDREN AND THEIR PARENTS

Illness and disability in children contradict our basic assumptions of life. Children are supposed to be vibrant, healthy, and have long lives ahead. Even the thought of a child suffering challenges all that we believe about the proper order of things, justice, and the essence of life. The prospect of one's child suffering and dying are almost unbearable. In fact, avoidance of the prospect of illness, suffering, and death in children is evidenced by the very limited attention given to the topic of pediatric suffering. Yet the Institute of Medicine reports that more than 50,000 children die each year from illness and disability in the United States (Institute of Medicine, 2002). The global numbers are staggering, particularly in underprivileged, war-torn countries.

Pediatrician Dr. Barbara Shapiro writes of suffering in children and their developmental differences. Children experience suffering similar to their developmental abilities, life experience, and understanding of illness and death. A child who is overwhelmed by the emotions of others and for whom the health-care environment is completely foreign may experience intense suffering despite the presence or absence of physical pain. Children may suffer—even more intensely than adults—when all that is familiar and secure disappears and is replaced by uncertainty and threat (Shapiro, 1996).

The suffering of an ill adolescent may be less associated with fear but related more to the losses stemming from illness. The loss of independence, of young adulthood, of romance and marriage, and of bodily integrity may all be factors. The painful venipuncture of a frightened 3 year-old is difficult to compare to the experience of a 17 year-old hospitalized in isolation with leukemia who is missing the homecoming dance. Both the 3 year-old and the 17 year-old experience suffering that transcends the physical injury. Both need support that is multidimensional and developmentally appropriate.

The suffering of the child resonates and often reverberates through the parents, grandparents, and siblings. A parent in a recent study described having a child diagnosed with cancer as " . . . having your child snatched from your arms and dangled over a river." She said her suffering intensified when the child's pain was poorly controlled and that it was like "being forced to watch your child fall into a river and drown" (Ferrell, Rhiner, Shapiro, and Dierkes, 1994). Siblings suffer tremendously as they feel challenged to protect their ill brother or sister, their parents, and their grandparents and as they face the loss of their sibling, often a best friend.

Illness often results in regression of development of children of all ages, particularly the adolescent. When faced with a life of chronic or terminal illness, adolescents often regress to earlier developmental levels and assume dependence on parents and seize the security of earlier childhood as they face the threat of serious illness or death.

Illness in any individual influences the entire family. In the case of children, the impact on multiple generations is even more profound. One mother said that her child's cancer "was as if someone threw a grenade in our living room," and that ". . . . we were a close family, but I'll tell you, cancer can kill a close family" (Ferrell, Rhiner, Shapiro, and Dierkes, 1994). Illness in children also impacts entire communities as schools and neighborhoods witness the illness or death of a child.

The research of Wolfe and colleagues (Wolfe et al., 2000) exposed the undertreatment of cancer pain in children through examination of the relationship of symptoms with suffering in children with cancer. Overall, 89% of the children experienced a great deal of suffering from at least one symptom, and 51% experienced three or more symptoms. Fatigue, pain, dyspnea, and poor appetite were the most commonly reported symptoms. Those children who died of a treatment-related complication suffered more symptoms than those who died of progressive disease. Wolfe has asserted that the suffering of children may be worse than that of adults because the parents and health-care providers are so aggressive in treating childhood illness or injury. Parents and health-care providers may avoid recognizing the pain or suffering of a child through "protective denial" and their hope for a miraculous healing of the child. There is often a spoken or unspoken belief that the child "will forget" the suffering or that all that has been endured will be "worth it" when the child recovers.

Similarly, children who know they may die may be less tolerant of the associated suffering than those who endure physical pain and isolation with the hope of becoming adults and reclaiming their threatened lives. A pediatric nurse shared her own anguish in caring for a 16 year-old girl whose HIV treatment had left her with multiple side effects, including obesity, chronic pancreatitis, discolored teeth, and skin lesions. The young woman spoke little of these physical effects but shared the suffering she experienced in missing out on all the adolescent social events and, most of all, the fear that she would not ever graduate, go to prom, drive, experience sexual intimacy, marry, or have children.

Suffering in children is often linked to physical pain, but it is very important to emphasize that children suffer psychologically, spiritually, and socially. The child's inability to control their own suffering is a severe insult and yet another insult to the child's desire for autonomy and control.

In literature, the search for meaning in illness among ill adults is a frequent topic. This search is also highly relevant for children and their parents. In our research related to children with cancer and their parents (Ferrell, Rhiner, Shapiro, and Dierkes, 1994), parents reported that children questioned why the illness or treatment had to be so bad. Parents most often questioned God for inflicting such unimaginable torture that caused the illness and pain in a child. As one parent said:

> I feel like I've been cheated with my kids. That's what I feel, and He knows it. I can't hide that. I ask Him a hundred times, 'Why are You doing this with my son?' An innocent child, you know. "Why [do] You have to put him through this pain? If You want to take him, just take him, and don't make him suffer like this.' I ask God that question a lot of times.

In this study, parents' suffering was often related to their inability to eradicate the child's suffering. One father described how it felt to be a successful professional in a business in which he controlled a company and a hundred employees. He would then leave work to come to the hospital and feel the devastation of having no control over his child's illness, treatment, pain, or suffering. In our study and others, one of the only comforting aspects reported by parents was to meet other parents of ill children. They would often meet late at night in waiting rooms after their exhausted children had fallen asleep, and they would share their experiences. These "communities of suffering" offer a deep, shared connection, and somehow in telling their stories to kindred spirits, their mutual suffering meets with some consolation as they have retreated to intense isolation from the world at large.

Another important observation in our research has been the divergent perspectives on faith between ill children and their parents. Children often rely intuitively on their faith, at whatever level of development, to endure suffering. Dying children speak of "going to heaven" or "being an angel with God," while their parents frequently question a God that would cause such circumstances. Although awareness may be internally comforting to the child nearing death, it may cause further anguish for parents when their child starts talking in such phrases. Parents also often wince at a child's discussion of heaven, which although comforting to the child, creates the anguishing reality that perhaps the child will soon die.

Parents may also cling to their faith, even after lashing out at what they perceive as a vengeful and unjust God. As one mother described, "[W]e still haven't adjusted to it, but on the other hand we have a firm faith, and we firmly believe God didn't want this to happen. I mean, He permitted it to happen, and we've just got to make—we've just got to make lemonade from lemons. We've just got to look at the half-cup theory, and look at it being half full, and then go on from there. But, we were very bitter, extremely bitter, and it was a true test of our faith initially. And now we accept it."

In the Pediatric ELNEC project, pediatric nurses were asked to define the concept "suffering." Table 3.5 includes examples of these definitions.

Interestingly, these pediatric nurses' definitions of suffering seemed rather depersonalized and abstract, and they generally did not refer to specific children or parents. However, when these nurses were asked to describe instances of pediatric suffering, they were able to provide profound examples, which are included in Table 3.6.

These nurses described pediatric suffering as the presence of unrelieved pain and the distress caused when children endured futile life-sustaining treatments. The nurses also described their own personal and moral suffering as a result of the children's experiences. At times, nurses see themselves as strong advocates for relief of the child's suffering, while at other times they feel impotent in their ability to relieve the suffering. It is also powerful to realize how their memories of these children's suffering and death remain so vivid even years or decades later.

Pediatric nurses in our survey were asked to describe their role in relieving suffering. They said they were primarily parent or child advocates, confronting physicians when pain was unrelieved or when futile care persisted. One nurse shared the experience of her own daughter's death and the care she received from her nurse colleagues.

> Sometimes nurses are the only support parents may receive. My daughter was in the PICU in the hospital where I worked. The nurses (even the ones who didn't know me) stood by me and supported me 100%. They allowed me to put my own daughter's clothes on her and uphold her dignity. They allowed my daughter's friends (four year-olds), whose parents felt it was appropriate, to see her. Her therapist was able to say her goodbyes. They let me hold her and sing to her and continue to be a mother. They allowed me to bathe her and dress her when she had died so I could see her left "pretty." They still keep in touch with me. They were my lifeline!

Table 3.5. Pediatric Nurses' Descriptions of the Term "Suffering"

It is a state where there is a disruption in the normalcy of one's world. The underlying conflict in suffering is pain, which can manifest in different realms: physical, psychosocial, spiritual, and financial. Suffering, if not addressed at any level can escalate to a state where the real world is seen in dismal light and colors.

I think most people associate pain with suffering, which I agree, but I want to write about the long-term grief process families experience and the suffering they experience along the way. Mom's and Dad's suffer when they are "left alone." Their child has died, their friends stop talking to them, relatives avoid the subject and everyone goes back to "normal life." The family has to find a new life to continue on.

Often resources are not available for counseling of a bereavement process. Everyone around you wants to put a "time-frame" on your grief (because they don't want to see you sad). It's almost as if you experience a second death: the death of yourself (the person you were) in the 1–3 years after your loss.

To feel the pain yourself, or to stand helplessly by as your loved one goes through it.

Suffering happens when our human drive to have meaning is impeded or unsupported or unacknowledged. Our own suffering can also be the wellspring of our compassion.

Suffering means more than physical pain; suffering is the torment felt deep inside a parent when their child is facing death, anger, guilt and fear, and questions of faith. The child can feel all those feelings. Also depending on age and level of understanding. The older child suffers with questions of "Why not me?"

Hopelessness and desperation—the feeling that there is no comfort possible for that person's particular distress. A person "suffering" seems to receive no relief and to be or feel very alone.

To suffer is to be without hope. Suffering can be physical, emotional, relational, or spiritual. To attempt to alleviate suffering is truly an art. It must be navigated. Our inclination is to navigate from our perspective. Rather it must arise from the patient and family. The greatest way we can help is to assist the family to clarify meaning and redefine hope. "Suffering" also stems from the fear of abandonment. Presence is a great intervention in reducing suffering.

To feel physical or emotional pain as a result of a chronic, terminal, or undiagnosed condition. To feel the pain yourself, or to stand helplessly by as your loved one goes through it.

Feeling powerless in an expected or unexpected situation that threatened the normal way of life. Unable to express your wishes and/or not have your wishes respected and carried out regarding your body, mind, and soul.

In the Pediatric ELNEC training, nurses reflected on being present for parents. One nurse described the nurse's primary function as agent of the ill child: "Nurses play a major role for those who are suffering. They are the eyes, ears, and hands of the patient. They are the advocates for the patient. They see what the patient needs; listen to the needs of the patient, and do what the patient cannot do for themselves or their families when they are suffering."

Table 3.6. Pediatric Nurses' Observations of Suffering

Physical Pain

A young girl had a non-operative, malignant tumor in her abdomen and rectum. Her father was a preacher and told her mother that if she (the mom) would only pray enough, the child would get better. Since they believed she would get better, they refused hospice or even nursing care at home. The child's pain worsened over the course of a few weeks, but the parents refused pain meds or care. The mother was in denial even as her child lay writhing and moaning in pain. We attempted to get a court order, but she died before it happened. I believe everyone suffered from this experience, especially the child. Mom, Dad, nurses, doctors, and social workers all suffered.

A child I took care of just the other night had burns to 25% of his body. During his dressing he was sedated with morphine, versed and ketamine. It took a while as you can only guess. I was in charge of the holding. Anyways, the ketamine wore off and he screamed out in pain. Praise was given to how well he was doing, but no further meds were given. Later on that night, he again needed his back redressed. I was in charge of the meds this time and whenever he woke up, more ketamine was given. What a difference it made for him and his family.

A 10-year-old girl with osteogenic sarcoma with recurrent disease screamed in pain, despite the continuous administration of morphine, right up until the last breath.

A 17-year-old male with terminal osteosarcoma would hit himself on the head to take away the real pain in his pelvis. His Mom brought him in this way. It took 2 days to adequately control his pain.

Futile Treatments/Unnecessary Procedures

I remember a 15-year-old boy with ALL relapse who died in February of this year. He was palliative since September 2005, but still receiving new chemo in hopes that his leukemia would surrender. He had intractable pain and suffering from various side effects/symptoms. The team (including R.N.'s) constantly changed his plan in order to help alleviate his suffering, but I don't think he ever stopped suffering. And I will always remember that.

Patient X, a 23-weeker, lived 105 days. He was always vented and outgrew his lungs. He went through a lot—PDL, multiple central line placements, intubations, blood draws. His parents deeply loved him and visited every day. They were repeatedly offered to have their son taken off the vent as his settings were so high—that any more would "blow up" his lungs. His parents refused, stating their son would decide when he would die, not them. We gave him pain meds and prayed his life would end quickly. It was very hard to see his grimacing face, clinched hands, and attempts to cry around his ET every time we did his care. His parents suffered too—watching him. They knew that they would suffer a great deal more if they "ended" his life, so they let him choose his own time.

The Anticipation of the Loss of a Child

The mom of a 1-year-old female given a terminal diagnosis. This mom is non-English speaking, from Mexico, having lost a son 10 years prior to admission. The son was 2 years old, ill since 7 months of age, and slowly failed to thrive. I cared for this patient for 12 months, until she died days prior to her second birthday of Duchene Muscular Dystrophy—now believed to be the cause of her brother's death 10 years ago in Mexico.

(*continued*)

Table 3.6. (continued)

Her mom meticulously cared for the patient, knowing she was going to die. The mom wore her suffering on her face—it told me "it is more difficult because I know what it's like losing a child."

I took care of an 18-month-old with an optic tumor (terminal). The father, who was a giant of a man, would come in to be with his daughter, pick her up and rock her, crooning and saying her name. He would cry softly for a long time. He knew his baby girl was dying.

In my experience as a hospice nurse, the situation that demonstrates suffering best was a mother whose son was admitted to our hospice program after he suffered a severe head injury/trauma at the hands of her fiancé. The child was a beautiful, happy, and healthy 1 year-old who was rendered unresponsive and with minimal brain activity. This mother experienced a terrible ordeal with suffering on all levels.

A recent ECMO patient case in which the patient was physically suffering. She exhibited signs of physical discomfort and pain. At the same time, the family was spiritually and emotionally suffering. They were devastated that their baby was not going to survive. It also caused them to question their religion. They did not understand why their God would give them a child only to take her away.

Children Suffering Because of Parents' Refusal to let go

I cared for a patient on maximum support for a condition which the medical team felt he would not recover from. The patient's mom refused to allow the team to discontinue support and he lived for several weeks while ethics meetings took place. The baby was on pain medication, but never appeared comfortable and was awake and agitated most of the time. He truly seemed to be suffering. I believe the mom was also suffering as she was isolated from the caregivers who felt a different course of action needed to be taken.

Children Blaming Themselves

The child who has experienced suffering tries to protect the parents from worrying or have them be sad about the situation. A 5-year-old boy gets up at 2 A.M., his mother found him on the bed. He has been praying for the protection of his parents. This child did not get informed that he is dying, but he knew it. Or the child will not say to the parents that he is in pain at all. But he opens his mouth if his mother gives him morphine because he does not want mom to worry.

Participants also saw the nurse as the key person to assess needs and coordinate interdisciplinary care. They witnessed suffering and called social workers, child psychologists, chaplains, or child-life specialists. Nurses were the "conductors of the orchestra." It is very important and encouraging to see that nurses recognize the importance of interdisciplinary care rather than feel that they alone can meet the child's and parents' needs.

Nurses also recognized that the greatest relief they could offer was *presence*. When asked what nurses do to relieve suffering in children and families, many offered simple but direct answers: "Be there," they said, "listen." One nurse wrote of her colleagues:

To me the nurses are like incredible quilts. They are comfort, protection, warmth, squares of the quilt in each function they perform—being parents themselves, administering drugs, emotionally supporting the families and children—too many roles to count . . . A conglomeration of patterns that make up the whole.

The suffering of nurses working in pediatrics was also voiced through narratives that described their dedication to continue working with seriously ill and dying infants and children even after years of cumulative loss and the emotional burden of witnessing suffering. One nurse captured the essence of nurses as simply "showing up".

Sometimes we can only witness. We cannot fix or do the work of creating meaning. This family responds to support, to ideas, to reframing, but ultimately they have to wrestle with the guilt themselves. We can provide a container, a holding environment of safety so they don't have to do this in isolation. We can keep showing up, even when it's messy and ragged and uncomfortable.

Because the idea of a sick or dying child is so against the natural order of life, parents cling to the hope of miraculous recovery. Nurses recognize their role in supporting these hopes, regardless of how unlikely a cure might be. One participant in our nursing education project wrote, "The nurse is the one person who has the opportunity and the responsibility to compassionately walk with the suffering family—advocating for the dignity of their child's life—thereby allowing the family to regain hope."

Pediatric nurses, as well as nurses in other contexts, did not directly cite Cassell's work, but the language in their narratives suggests that they are familiar with his concept of suffering as a threat to the intactness or wholeness of a person. Many nurses have described their role as helping those who are suffering to become whole. Most nurses also acknowledge the importance of attention to physical, psychological, social, and spiritual needs.

Pediatric nurses recognize the "conspiracy of silence," in which children often do not tell their parents about their pain and suffering. Parents hide their grief from the children. Siblings are protected. Grandparents hold the silent vigil, consumed with the enormity of the suffering of all they love. The nurses often see themselves as the central person that each suffering person can communicate with honestly. Children tell nurses things they would hide from their parents; siblings ask nurses what is really happening; parents and grandparents share their rarely articulated recognition that an ill child may not survive. The conspiracy of silence breeds more suffering. The long-term impact on siblings is considerable, and nurses have much to contribute to the bereavement support of all involved when they can break the conspiracy of silence and foster honest communication.

Nurses recognize the challenge of maintaining a healthy boundary between their role as a clinician and their role as a compassionate person. They see themselves as the professional who spends the most time with children and families, the coordinator of care, and the interpreter of needs. Nurses have described many specific tasks, such as identifying the sources of suffering, advocating for needs, and providing information; as one nurse described, "Sometimes the most profound thing a nurse can do is to become a familiar support person, the 'clinical friend.' "

Nurses clearly feel accountable for meeting the child and family needs as far as they are able. One nurse defined her role: "To be available, to be present, to be an advocate, to know the resources available and how to access them, to listen, to realize the buck stops here—find help for the patient however I can." Pediatric nurses consistently describe themselves as "on the frontlines." One nurse wrote:

> I have always thought the clichés nurses use such as "don't die on my shift," have always compelled me to volunteer to take care of the dying patient, knowing it would be painful, uncomfortable, and I would feel inadequate. Yet my heart was meant to be there. It is my passion and my calling. I have taught grief courses and one of the most important messages I pass on is "It isn't a curse or bad day or why me?" when you are assigned the dying patient. It is an honor what you do and say to that person or baby. If we can't save their life, it's the most important job the nurse can do. We can give of ourselves to that family because they will remember every detail and memory of the care that we gave.

The nurse's "frontline" is also being the clinician who is willing to honestly discuss the child's declining condition when other professionals, particularly physicians, are often hesitant to do so. Nurses see themselves as the accessible person to answer the frequent question of "What's going to happen next?"

THE CONTEXT OF GERIATRICS

The suffering of elderly people has many unique characteristics. For many aging individuals, physical discomfort is much less a concern than the psychosocial consequences of living a long life. The 90-year-old man who has outlived his wife by 10 years is now limited in physical function, sight, and memory, and who has had the unfortunate experience of having buried two of his own children, knows suffering on many levels.

Professional and lay literature has often depicted elderly life as that portrayed in "The Golden Girls," suggesting that "70 is the new 50" and that "aging well" can prevent the negative consequences of growing old. Although these media messages are appealing, aging in even the most ideal circumstances offers profound life changes and is accompanied by multiple losses (Potter, 2006). To live fully and to love is to ultimately experience loss and to face mortality, whether at 70 or 100.

The psychological work of growing old can be immense. Elderly people are letting go of all aspects of their lives. They may have a spouse and many life-long friends who are also facing the same challenges of aging. They may be seeking a sense of life completion and searching intently for meaning in their lives as they review the years that have passed by. The elderly may also suffer from a loss of cognitive capacity and physical independence, which becomes a part of their daily living (Ersek and Wilson, 2003).

Nurses in geriatric settings must learn to distinguish between normal sadness and clinical depression (Pasacreta, Minarik, and Nield-Anderson, 2006). Their patients not only have the intense loss of relationships and identities but also the loss of privacy, dignity, and intrusion that often accompany dependence. The experiences of the elderly and their associated suffering are influenced greatly by their cumulative life experiences. In a previous study conducted at the City of Hope, we evaluated QOL issues for women with breast cancer. We held separate focus groups of young, middle-aged, and older women, because we recognized that the issues for a newly married 38-year-old woman might be very different from an 85-year-old woman. In the focus group consisting of older women, one patient with advanced disease and an extremely brutal treatment regimen seemed to be coping exceptionally well. When questioned, the woman replied that it was "*only*" breast cancer, and she went on to describe the losses of her life: a husband from divorce and a home taken by a hurricane, to name only two. Although she "only" had breast cancer, she became intensely sad when she described how she had lost a son to cancer the previous year. As she shared what it meant to outlive one's own child, her suffering seemed most intense.

The suffering of elders often is felt intensely by their family. Alzheimer's disease is now a common example of the distress in geriatrics as this disease becomes more prevalent in our aging population. Sons and daughters witness the slow but obvious decline in parents who change from independent and supportive to dependent and unable to manage personal care or make simple decisions (Collins, Liken, King, and Kokinakis, 1993; Talerico, 2003).

Suffering may be expressed in a sentiment such as, "Why am I still here?" A 93-year-old woman who had "buried three husbands," lost a leg to complications of diabetes, and was blind never complained about her physical symptoms, dependence, or list of medical diagnosis. Instead she asked the staff "When will the Good Lord come to His senses and take me home?" While she is pleasant to staff and other residents, she confides to the nurses that each morning when she awakens and realizes she's still alive, suffering overcomes her.

Nurses also express their distress in watching lives that go on too long. When elders endure life-prolonging treatments, especially when their expressed wishes are ignored, the moral distress of nurses is even more pronounced. Nurses who work in long-term care settings witness residents who were once active participants in social activities decline to the point of being confined to bed with limited ability to express even the most basic needs. Table 3.7 includes narratives of suffering shared by nurses in relation to their elderly patients.

The issues of isolation and loneliness are bluntly expressed in these stories, which also depict the essential role of the nurse in diminishing suffering. In the first three examples, the nurse's primary act was to be present, to offer human touch, and to hear the voice of the sufferer. The fourth example is illustrative of the "unwinding" of a life. As the aging physical body declines, psychological and physical sequelae follow, resulting in little control. Nurses compassionately respond to elderly patients with dedication to preserving dignity. Nurses take great pride in being able to orchestrate the final weeks or months of life such that a dignified life is mirrored in a dignified end of life.

SHARED SUFFERING: THE SUFFERING
OF FAMILY CAREGIVERS

The patient contexts presented earlier have referred to the shared suffering within families across diseases and settings. Family members often become a reflection of the patient's suffering as that reflection is cast back onto the patient. Suffering within families is both an intensely individual experience as each son, daughter, or spouse responds within their relationship as well as a collective, shared suffering experience of family (Hickman, Tilden, and Tolle, 2004).

Most literature focuses on individual caregivers, such as partners of women with breast cancer or adult children caring for a parent with Alzheimer's Disease. Limited attention has been given to the family as a system or to the collective suffering among family members. The strong association

Table 3.7. Geriatric Nurses' Observations of Suffering

When I was a new nurse, I worked in a nursing home on a subacute floor. I was getting a report from the previous nurse who informed me that one of my patients was dying. He had been without food/drink for 17 days, weighed about 60 lbs, did not have family. He had morphine as needed for pain, but none had been used, because the nurse said he was "fine." When I arrived at his room, this nurse had followed me in. His door had been closed! He began to cry and the sounds he made were not even human. I had never heard anything like it. I introduced myself and said "You seem to be in a lot of pain, where does it hurt?" With the same animal-like cry he said, "Everywhere." I told him I would get some morphine. He began crying again, saying, "All I want is someone to lay down with me." The nurse who had given me report turned to me and said, "You'd be fired if you ever did anything like that." Well, that's all I needed to hear because it reinforced what I needed to do. With my nursing license one week old, I got some morphine and went back to my patient's room, and after giving the morphine, I laid next to him for a few minutes. I held his hand and told him that it would be okay and reassured him that he was not alone. He thanked me with the last bit of strength he had and died peacefully within the next few hours. This to me was human suffering—all he needed was human touch. How simple!

A patient with advanced dementia was lying in bed, moaning continuously. I asked her if she was in pain, if she was uncomfortable, if "anything hurt," and if she had any discomfort. She replied "no" to all of my questions. I asked, "if nothing hurts, then why do you keep moaning?" She replied, "Oh honey, it's my soul that hurts."

A patient I had in hospice was restless. He had an expression of fear on his face. A glaze in his eye as if he wanted to talk but didn't know who to trust. After a while, I got to know him. He was dying and he had not been to church in some time for one reason or another. We talked further and he said he believed in God, that He had died for his sins. After that, he let a chaplain in. They prayed. He renewed his faith and was at peace. At peace with life and death.

This was a lady in her 80s. She had always been young for her age. She loved to go anywhere, anytime. Various members of her family took her out. Then she developed bulbar Amyotrophic Lateral Sclerosis. As the disease progressed, she became unable to talk, drooled constantly, and had to have a gastric feeding tube. She stated she could no longer enjoy life. She ended up in a skilled nursing facility. Became increasingly dyspneic and anxious. The dyspnea and anxiety progressed to being out of control. It took several hours to get it under control. She died a peaceful death.

of "pain and suffering" can be applied to family caregivers because caring for a patient in pain is an extreme case of suffering for the family caregiver as witness. In an exploration of the impact of pain on family caregivers, pain is seen as a metaphor for the status of the illness (Ferrell, Rhiner, Cohen, and Grant, 1991). Seeing a patient in pain signifies that the patient is worse and will die soon. Table 3.8 lists the words used by family caregivers to describe their loved one's pain and subsequent suffering.

The suffering of family members themselves is cited in various literature (Ferrell, 2001; Ferrell, Ervin, Smith, Marek, and Melancon, 2002; Price

Table 3.8. Word Descriptors Used by Caregivers to Describe the Pain of Their
Loved Ones

Aching	Hurting	Sore
Agonizing	Inconceivable	Spastic
Agony	Intense	Squeezing
Bad	Intermittent	Stabbing
Burning	Itching	Strong
Constant	Miserable	Tense
Continuous	Overwhelming	Terrible
Cramping	Pressure	Throbbing
Debilitating	Pulling	Tightness
Exasperating	Pushing	Tingling
Excruciating	Radiating	Traveling
Extreme	Searing	Unbearable
Horrendous	Severe	Uncomfortable
Horrible	Sharp	Uncontrollable
Hot		

Adapted with permission from Ferrell, B.R., M. Rhiner, M.Z. Cohen, and M. Grant. (1991). Pain as
a metaphor for illness part I: Impact of cancer pain on family caregivers. *Oncology Nursing Forum.*
18:1303–1309.

1996). Sherman and Reuben (1998) studied elderly caregivers and described their "reciprocal suffering," whereas Boland and Sims (1996) used
the term "solitary journey" to describe the 24-hour-a-day, monumental task
of providing home care. Lederberg (1998) articulated a concern for the
health of family caregivers as they took on the physical and emotional
burdens of the patient and became at high risk for decline of their own
health as "second order patients" (Lederberg, 1998). Burdens imposed by
the patient, such as depending on others for bathing or feeding, are also
often the greatest sources of distress to those same patients. The ill person
often wishes for death to ease the burden on caregivers (Wilson, Curran,
and McPherson, 2005).

The role of caregiver as witness to illness is described by Horowitz and
Lanes (1992):

> Being witness has a peculiar property of being separate from the
> action, yet at the same time fully engaged. There is sympathy and
> empathy, resentment and compassion. Often the patient's pain or
> distress is indirectly felt, transformed, vividly imagined, or distorted
> by thinking it is much worse than it really is. Witnesses are afraid
> for the patient and themselves as they, too, face change, while
> wishing for a return to normalcy.

Although patients and families may hold similar beliefs about pain, family caregivers tend to have a higher degree of emotional distress associated

with observing pain in their loved one (Miaskowski, Zimmer, Barrett, Dibble, and Wallhagen, 1997; Ferrell, Taylor, Sattler, Fowler, and Cheyney, 1993). In caring for their loved one, it is the sense of helplessness that increases the suffering in the caregiver. Table 3.9 offers narratives from such family caregivers.

One of the most important contributions to nursing literature related to family caregiving was provided by Dr. Betty Davies (Davies, 2006). Davies conducted interviews of family caregivers to understand their perspectives of the patient's decline in cancer. She described the process whereby caregivers realized the patient was not living with cancer but dying from it. Her works identified seven dimensions of families' experiences of seeing the patient "fade away," which included redefining, burdening, struggling with paradox, contending with change, searching for meaning, living day by day, and preparing for death (Davies, 2006, 547). The process is not linear; rather, the phases are interrelated. Davies identified key nursing interventions to support families through these phases and emphasized the importance of listening and recognizing that the spiritual pain of losing a loved one cannot be removed but can be witnessed and supported.

How a family caregiver deals with observing pain and suffering in a loved one is significantly influenced by the nature of his/her relationship with the ill person (Ferrell, 2001). Therefore, providing support for family caregivers requires an understanding of the specific psychological, social, and spiritual distresses of the caregiver (Borneman et al., 2003). The assessment of needs of the family caregiver becomes a common task of the nurse, as it is the nurse who has interacted most with patients and their family caregivers, allowing him/her the ability to direct patients and their family caregivers toward the appropriate support services. It is the nurse at the frontline of care who best understands how to move a family caregiver from a sense of helplessness to a sense of helpfulness. Understanding culture and ethnicity are vital to being of service to diverse cultures and, more specifically, in respecting religious heritage (Lartey, 2003).

Recent contributions to nursing scholarship in this area are seen in the doctoral research by Mary Jo Prince-Paul (Prince-Paul, 2006). Her two studies directly related to suffering will be reviewed in some detail. She sought to examine the applicability of Ferrell and Grant's QOL Conceptual Model with patients suffering from advanced cancer at the end of life. This model has primarily been used in the cancer survivorship population. Because the social well-being domain of the QOL has been largely untapped through empirical investigation, from the end-of-life perspective, descriptive research was conducted to explore its meaning, constituents, and predictive ability on the QOL at the end of life (QOLEOL). In addition, close personal relationships and the communication between these relationships—specifically

Table 3.9. Family Caregivers: The Burden of Care

Home Care—Responsibilities and Exhaustion

I'm afraid to leave her alone. She might fall or have an angina attack. I feel guilty if I go out for any length of time. She tells me to go and then asks me why I've been so long. I've taken over the woman's work in the home, cooking and cleaning. She has too much pain and is too sick to do it.

Home Care—Watching Deterioration

Each day sucks for me, hard to get up. I'm just watching him waste away, only his spirit left. It's so hard. I just don't like to see it happen. Hard to watch. Even though we have wonderful friends I'm the one who sits and watches him each day.

I've been floating on that long dark ocean all on my own for the past month. He's not in pain, just fading away. The doctor says make him more comfortable. I don't know what that means.

Home Care—Own Needs not Being Met

It's so hard. I'm not a nurturer. That's why I didn't have children. I have no time to do anything for myself. He gets angry with me. I'm separated from my art. I always said that would kill me. I'm dying piece by piece.

My husband's world view is narrowed to focus on his immediate needs and TV. My needs and the children's are much wider. I deeply care for him, but the strain is great.

Home or Hospital as the Place of Care?

I want him to be at home when he dies but what am I going to do? I want him to die at home but I don't know what to do when he talks about his funeral clothes, what he wants to wear, about cremation.

I can nurse him to life. I cannot nurse him to death. He is lost to me now.

Loss of Life As It Was

I can't believe all of this. Eight months ago she was well, we were having a good time. Now she is lying there, her eyes open, hallucinating. She didn't sleep last night. She lay there talking to herself. She didn't seem to be in pain.

Loss of Hope

I've given up hope. I cry no more. Once I learned he had a brain tumor nothing was left. It's awful to live without hope. I wish it was over already for both him and for me. He has lost his spirit. It's no fun for him watching family members catering to him, being scared because of him.

Loss of the Person I Knew

I felt an intense sadness as I looked at her. Something vital in her has been eroded by drugs, by pain, by the disease.

Wanting Death to Come Soon

I feel guilty for saying this, but I wish it was over.

(continued)

Table 3.9. (continued)

We're all psyched up for her to die. Psyched up that she's not going to make it. If she does, it'll be a miracle. I don't want her to go on living with all this pain. If she goes under I don't want her to be resuscitated. Her spirits are nil. She's in and out of a trance.

Adapted with permission from Coyle, N. (1996). Suffering in the first person: Glimpses of suffering through patients' and family narratives. In *Suffering*, ed. B.R. Ferrell, 29–64. Sudbury, MA: Jones & Bartlett.

the verbal exchange of gratitude, love, and forgiveness—were also investigated. Relationship affirmation, the communicative act and process between a person with a life-limiting disease and a significant other addressing some or all of the critical components of love, gratitude, and forgiveness, was a new concept that was also proposed by the author. Because of the lack of empirical knowledge about the importance of personal relationships at the end of life and knowledge about relationship affirmation, progress in developing theoretical insight about this concept requires empirical investigation. Prince-Paul postulated that if knowledge about the meaning of social well-being at the end of life from the perspective of the terminally ill patient with cancer is gained, it will broaden the understanding of QOLEOL, specifically contributing to our understanding of the importance and meaning of close, personal relationships.

This hermeneutic, phenomenological investigation by Prince-Paul, aiming to understand the meaning of social well-being at the end of life from the dying person's perspective, identified six themes: meaning of relationships with family, friends, and coworkers; meaning of relationships with God or a Higher Power; loss and gains of role functions; love; gratitude; and lessons on living. All eight terminally ill participants with cancer in Prince-Paul's study revealed the heightened importance of maintaining close, personal relationships but also the need to express the importance of these relationships through the communicative acts of love and gratitude. Additionally, many of the respondents focused on their relationships with others that had been "difficult" and described them as "closer" as a result of the cancer experience. Most respondents acknowledged how their roles had changed within the context of their illness and their relationships with others. Although there were differences in how each role was defined and how it functioned, all participants expressed the desire to maintain current roles with some sense of "normalcy." Most importantly, and probably most informative to the potential shared composition of the social and spiritual domains of the QOLEOL, was the participants' discussion of a relationship with God or a higher Power as a close, personal relationship. All participants believed that this relationship, defined as human or existential, was strengthened by the cancer experience. These findings laid the groundwork for a subsequent quantitative investigation by Prince-Paul on *"Relationships among Communicative Acts, Social Well-Being, and Spiritual Well-Being on the Quality of Life at the End of Life."*

This cross-sectional, descriptive correlational study sought to explore associations among close, personal relationships in 50 newly admitted hospice patients with a cancer diagnosis and the domains of QOLEOL. Utilizing the three predictors of social well-being, spiritual well-being, and communicative acts on QOL at the end of life (measured by a single-item indicator), the overall model revealed that spiritual well-being was the greatest predictor of overall QOL. Social well-being offered the second largest contribution to overall QOL.

Fifty-two percent of the participants in the study indicated a "complete" opportunity to express the words "thank you" and "I love you" to those important to them. However, the subjects had particular difficulty in responding to the question about forgiveness. Despite a great deal of research in the social science literature regarding forgiveness, it has not received systematic investigation in the end-of-life population. Although hospice clinicians have suggested that forgiveness has important therapeutic value, it may not be as generally relevant as once believed. Clinicians may have associated the importance of facilitating forgiveness with the few situations where there were serious, unresolved conflicts and relational hurt and, subsequently, may have assigned a degree of importance and need to this concept. Although these intrapersonal processes have been postulated in the general population, further investigation is needed to provide conceptual clarity and valid measurement in the end-of-life population. Just as grief is a *process*, so may be forgiveness, and therefore it may not be part of the communicative acts concept.

Prince-Paul's work provides an increased understanding of how to identify patients and families with relationship issues as key to effective end-of-life clinical practice. This is important work as nurses need appropriate tools to facilitate conversation and communication among the patients, families, significant others, and physicians. Before designing and testing intervention strategies and tools, we must first gain a better understanding and empirical confirmation of the proposed elements of relationship affirmation and the effect of the specific communicative acts.

An example of valuable nursing research in progress to address the future of family caregiving in our society is the doctoral research of Polly Mazanec, R.N., N.P., a doctoral candidate at Case Western University in Cleveland. Her dissertation is, "Distant Caregiving for a Parent with Advanced Cancer" (2007).

Because of today's changing society and global workplace, many adult children find themselves in the role of distant caregiver for a parent with advanced disease. Distant caregiving, the experience of providing instrumental and emotional support to an ill loved one who lives a long distance from the caregiver, is on the rise. More than seven million Americans are distant caregivers and the number is expected to grow as baby boomers and their parents age. Unlike previous generations in which adult children cared for parents in their own homes and/or communities, today's distant caregivers of parents are struggling with the demands of caregiving from a distance and often are doing it alone. They may lack social support from nearby family members and may be juggling multiple roles and responsibilities that make caregiving demands even more challenging.

Although much is known about the needs of local caregivers, there is almost no research on distant caregiving and the lasting impact—physical and emotional—on both distant caregivers and patients. Intervention studies are nonexistent. Although data from local caregivers can be applied to distant caregivers; however, distant caregivers are potentially at greater risk for caregiver burden and suffering related to limited access to resources, education, and support.

Mazanec's study is designed to identify the effects of distance on the caregiving experience and the extent to which the appraisal of the caregiving experience influences caregiver outcomes of anxiety, depression, and distress. Research on the distant caregiving experience will lay the foundation for future nursing intervention studies for this growing population of caregivers.

COMMON THREADS ACROSS CONTEXTS OF SUFFERING

The contexts selected for this chapter illustrate suffering across various patient experiences. Nurses in all settings encounter instances of suffering that share many similar but unique dimensions. Nurse researchers employing qualitative methods have explored many patient and family experiences that have been ignored previously in the biomedical paradigm of illness.

An example of nursing scholarship that has illuminated suffering is the book by Madjar and Walton, titled *Nursing and the Experience of Illness* (1999). This book presents several phenomenological studies that describe patient experiences of illness in contexts such as schizophrenia, chronic pain, and chronic leg ulcers. In the chapter "On Living with Schizophrenia," Walton illustrates the suffering of mental illness as "a sentence as well as a diagnosis" and a condition that is cruel, feared, and socially isolated. This work describes instances where research and medical care have focused on the tissue pathology but ignored the person. This text and others that explore human perspectives of illness cite Kleinman's definition of illness as "the innately human experience of symptoms and suffering" (Kleinman, 1988, 3). These authors point to the important issue that in mental illness, there are often no outward signs of disease. Phenomenological inquiry that identifies the internal struggles and experiences of mental illness are vital.

A common thread in the discussion of suffering is the importance of nursing presence and attentive listening. This is challenging for busy nurses in demanding environments. *Presence* is far more than being physically available or offering expert listening skills. True presence is a sacred act. It is transformative for the nurse as well as for the patient or family member. The theologian Henri Nouwen has written extensively on caring relationships and his writing is relevant to nursing and to this issue of presence. Nouwen wrote, "Compassion can never coexist with judgment because judgment creates the distance, the distinction, which prevents us from really being with the other" (Nouwen, 1991, 35).

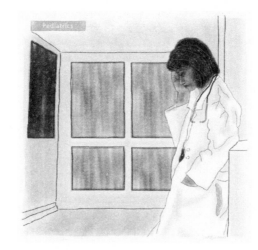

CHAPTER 4 ❧

The Suffering of Nurses

The previous chapters have addressed nurses' perspectives of patient and family suffering within specific contexts. There is also an association between the nurse's own suffering and the suffering he or she witnesses in others. There is often an inseparable relationship between the suffering person and the suffering of those professionals who witness suffering while providing care. This relationship can be close and intense, and each party is vulnerable to the other. At times, the nurse's own suffering may be a result of his or her interpretation that the patient is suffering; however, the patient's actual experience may be quite different. There is always the need to step back and ask, "Whose suffering am I experiencing? Is it my own or is it the patient's? Whose values are at stake here? Are they my own or are they the patient's?"

This chapter is devoted to the suffering of nurses. The powerful words in the previous chapters describing the suffering of people facing serious illness illustrate the daily work of nurses. These moving narratives are the very ordinary or, perhaps better stated, "extraordinary" work of nurses. Each of the patients described in the previous chapters are single faces but represent likely hundreds of patients cared for each year by a single nurse and thousands of suffering patients over one nurse's professional career.

At one of our end-of-life care training courses, a nurse said that her first year as a hospice nurse coincided with the annual memorial service for all of the patients who had died that year in their program. At first she was honored when she was asked to participate. Each nurse was called forward and asked to read the names of all their primary patients who had died. As she sat waiting for her turn, she began to feel a monumental weight on her shoulders. She looked at her list and realized she had been responsible for the care of 70 patients in the final days of their lives. Seventy lives had ended, 70 families had grieved. She asked herself if she had done enough to relieve their pain. She wondered how the families were doing.

This memorial ritual and the nurse's feelings associated with participation are a poignant example of the work of nursing. Nurses working in an ICU, a NICU, on an oncology unit, or in an ED come to work each day, aware that they will certainly witness suffering and that they are very likely to also witness death.

In *The Rebirth of the Clinic: An Introduction to Spirituality in Health Care* (2006), Daniel Sulmasy, M.D., emphasizes the importance of recognizing health-care providers' suffering if we are to tend to the suffering of patients and families. Sulmasy describes caring professionals as being in a relationship with the recipients of their care. He also wrote of the delicate balance of caring professionalism and compassionate presence:

> Neither is it a cold and unfeeling distance, however, or an objectification of the patient as a way of coping with his or her predicament. The patient deserves more than an automaton dispensing technology. The patient also deserves more than a weepy mess for a doctor or nurse. The burned-out health care professional helps no one. I am recommending that the health care professional recognize the unique vulnerability of the patient, ever mindful of the special vulnerability that comes from being one who truly gives *care*. (Sulmasy, 2006, 40)

Breitbart (2002) and Chochinov (2006) have addressed patients' search for meaning in their illness. Nurses also seek meaning in their work to sustain their ability to offer *presence* amidst suffering. In 1999, Fall-Dickson and Rose explored the stresses of oncology nurses and their search for meaning. They found that oncology nurses constantly worked to manage their patients' treatment-related side effects, a task that often proved difficult and caused distress for the staff. Some nurses described great angst and frustration when they experienced a lack of recognition and support for their diligence. On the other hand, the investigators found that nurses both derived a sense of purpose as well as developed close relationships with patients and families under conditions of great stress.

In struggling to find a delicate balance between continuing to do the work that health-care professionals do in the midst of the often discouraging diagnoses of the patient, Greg Sachs, M.D., recalls a poignant experience while treating a patient. Mrs. Smith was a 78-year-old woman whose chart listed her diagnoses as dementia, pressure sores, incontinence, diabetes, anemia, malnutrition, and multiple fractures. In the process of examining a hip sore, he arrives at an epiphany:

. . . I saw no organisms, the wound looked clean, and there was a strange clearness in the center of the crater. I took a deep breath and looked again at the ulcer . . . I noted movement within the sore. This time the movement paralleled my own motions. I moved closer and peered deeper into the cavity. Right in the center, in the deepest portion of the wound, I saw my own reflection staring back at me.

. . . Seeing oneself in a pressure sore is a stark and frightening vision, disturbing on many levels. In addition to the grotesque wound and personal reflection, it seemed to mirror the topsy-turvy medical care given to many such patients. Mrs. Smith came from a hospital where she received mechanical ventilation for a respiratory arrest suffered when she was hypoglycemic . . . Yet she lay long enough without being turned for all the tissue between her skin and bones to necrotize.

It is sad that somewhere in the course of a dementing process Mrs. Smith lost many of the characteristics that most of us associate with meaningful adult human life. It is sadder still that she received medical treatment that forgot about her as a human being.

It is fitting to have seen myself literally within Mrs. Smith and now to carry a vivid memory of her within me. It is a sharp reminder that I am always inside patients like Mrs. Smith and that they are always inside of me; all of us are a part of the human community, no matter how demented, contracted, or incontinent. Debilitated and dependent patients need us to reach out and care for them most when we are starting to push them away. It is our distancing of ourselves from these people that is the true dehumanizing act. (Sachs, 1988, 2145)

What Sachs offers is of great importance to the struggle of nurses trying to find meaning in their roles.

The ethical and moral experiences of oncology nurses also deserve discussion. O'Connor (1996) collected surveys from 70 oncology nurses, including narratives about their experiences in clinical situations in which they experienced ethical or moral dilemmas. The results of the survey described the suffering not only of patients with cancer but also of nurses. The nurses' experiences reflected a care perspective focused on principles such as protecting patient autonomy and the importance of truth-telling. Key themes from the analysis of the surveys included suffering, secrets, and struggle.

Steeves, Cohen, and Wise (1994) used a phenomenological approach to study 38 oncology nurses and their perceptions of the meaning of their work. Three roles were identified by the nurses, including maintaining the values of the organization through activities, such as monitoring the patients; participating in patients' experiences by being there for them, including during their last moments; and reconciling health-care values and patient experiences by truth-telling. Nurses in this study reported feelings of isolation in their work and the burdens of observing and experiencing suffering.

Oncology nurse researchers Dr. Marlene Cohen and Dr. Barbara Sarter (Cohen and Sarter, 1992) conducted one of the most in-depth explorations of suffering that reflects the suffering experienced by nurses. These scholars suggest that the relief of suffering is the essence of oncology nursing:

> . . . being on the front lines of a war against death, disfigurement, and intense human suffering. It requires the performance, prioritization, and coordination of multiple complex tasks. It involves handling frequent, unexpected crises, both physiologic and psychological. It carries the rewards of reversing a fatal illness, balanced by the ever-present reality of death. Working with patients with cancer requires constant vigilance in monitoring for sudden problems and life-threatening errors. The cancer nurse's empathy is sharpened by the awareness that "this could be me or my loved one." Finally, working with patients with cancer means "being there" for people in their most private moments of suffering and responding to the heights and depths of their responses to this suffering. (Cohen and Sarter, 1992, 1485)

The setting of oncology is the most cited with regard to nurses' suffering, given the prevalence of pain and death associated with cancer. There are many other contexts of nurses' suffering, and with the exception of a small percentage of nurses whose work is focused exclusively on prevention or wellness, all nurses encounter suffering in daily practice.

Table 4.1 includes geriatric nurses' descriptions of patient experiences with suffering. These narratives of caring for older people suggest that suffering in the elderly may come from simply living longer than the patient wants to live. On the contrary, in oncology narratives, death is often perceived as coming too soon. In each situation, nurses have their own emotional responses to these suffering patients.

In ICU settings (Table 4.2), nurses also experience the distress of working in the highest of technological and often most dehumanized en-

Table 4.1. Geriatric Nurses' Descriptions of Patient Suffering and Their
Own Responses

Geriatric patient with complete renal failure. The patient became confused over the last
few months but prior to becoming so had told nursing and his health-care agent he didn't
want dialysis. His agent disagreed and signed consent for dialysis anyway. This was very
frustrating for me. I felt angry because my hands were tied.

92-year-old woman who had a great quality of life before she had a disabling stroke. The
patient could have been spared the discomfort of the procedure. Medicare could have
been spared the cost of the procedure with better communication.

A 72-year-old female was semi-comatose and was being dialyzed. The nurses felt horrible at inflicting pain on the patient in the process of caring for her. Most of staff voiced
anger at an "absent" family that would let her suffer and prolong the dying process.

An 89-year-old man who had multiple symptoms and no quality of life. His wife of 60
years, however, wanted "everything done." When my patient coded we were obligated to
start cardiopulmonary resuscitation. With the first compression came a sound I shall never
forget—that of bones breaking. My patient died—and with so little dignity! I had my belief
reaffirmed that day that there are worse things than death. I became aware of the importance of educating patients and families so that they are able to make informed choices,
and when appropriate to reassure them that letting go can be the greatest gift of love.

It was frustrating and very sad that the wife was not able to follow her husband's wishes
and that the family is not ready to let go and talk about their loss and eventual death of
the husband. For the nurses at the bedside who care for the patient 24 hours a day and
see that his dying is only prolonged and that his suffering causes great distress.

Mrs. Z is a 66-year-old woman with a diagnosis of pancreatic cancer. She was diagnosed
approximately 1 year ago and underwent multiple chemo regimens. The most recent
was 10 weeks ago, and she developed severe dehydration requiring hospitalization. The
cost of this treatment is very expensive—$5,000 per month—the machine is $22,000.
Patient calls me "the torturer" and "Nurse Ratchet."

My patient was a 98-year-old lady who was not eating. The daughters had medical
power of attorney and wanted a nasogastric tube placed for feeding. Their reason was
that they had heard their mother say she wanted to live to be 100 years old. I assisted the
nurse who attempted to put in the tube. The patient began to cry as we attempted to
pass the tube. The other nurse decided to stop trying because it was causing the patient
distress. The nurse was acting on behalf of the patient and respecting her wishes not to
eat. However, it felt as though we were helpless/powerless because the physician was
doing whatever the daughters wanted. We had no "voice." We will continue to speak up
on behalf of our patients. It can be very discouraging and it sometimes seems like we may
never make a difference.

vironments. They must somehow manage the intense stress from the constant attempts to save lives, which is often followed only moments later by
the need to stand witness to medically futile care that continues long beyond
any hope for meaningful survival. The words in Table 4.2 illustrate the
powerful emotions of nurses as they describe "violent acts," "torture," and

Table 4.2. Critical Care Nurses' Descriptions of Suffering

When I worked in the NICU, many infants were just "pounded into the ground" in an effort to keep them alive. They died horrible, painful, protracted deaths. It is tremendously demeaning to be out of control yourself—being made to do cruel and tormenting interventions "because you are ordered to do them." It diminishes physicians and nurses to do these violent acts. Just because a family is out of control is no justification for medical staff. I worry that as a people we are losing sight of the futility we are willing to inflict on our patients.

Patient did not have a single functioning organ system. Patient's family was adamant we continue all aggressive treatment per their religious beliefs; they could not withdraw support. Palliative consult clearly identified these beliefs, clarified family's understanding and perception of patient's wishes . . . This case revealed to me the impact of seeing futile cases—at least quantitative—and how it affects the perspective of the nurses caring for these patients. This experience pointed out also the importance of all four areas—medical, psychological, social, and spiritual.

The 8-year-old patient coded three times in the last 48 hours of her life. Finally her aunt asked, "Why are you bringing her back?" No one could answer her except to say, "Policy." Finally, that aunt said after #3, "Don't torture that baby again." The staff got a social worker up to help the aunt speak with the doctors. I was horrified at the whole thing . . . I kept asking God to take her, it was time. God tried but the hospital staff wouldn't let go because of "policy."

The patient and her family were very religious, and I think that played a huge part in their decisions. They really believed God would help . . . Her leukemia returned . . . Her family continued to want everything done. She went to the ICU several times with infection and bleeding. We always had to keep a restraint on her because she had no sense of her limitations and fell if she were not restrained. She ended up in terrible emotional distress and pain at times. Her family avoided do-not-resuscitate discussions and hospice. This woman's last few months of life seemed to be full of suffering, and she coded and died in ICU without her family with her.

This patient was admitted to the ICU for abdominal surgery. A code was called for him. As I arrived in his room, the team was ready to shock him. I knew it was time for him to die. He had told me he was ready to die. Since there was no "do not resuscitate" order, the code was to proceed. I told the team he did not want this. I had to leave the room. His body recovered from this first insult and he remained in ICU for two more months until he slowly became septic and his body shut down and he died a slow, pitiful death. I felt very unable to help advocate for the patient. I felt very disempowered. It was a violation of my own beliefs about death and dignity.

---

feeling "disempowered." Technology such as ventilator support, dialysis, or chemotherapy may prolong life but may also greatly diminish QOL. The goals and values of patient and family may somehow get lost, and available technology, rather than goals of care, becomes the driving force of care.

By surveying nurses across a range of settings, including inpatient, ICU, ER, hospice, and long-term care, nurses' moral distress in witnessing this type of "futile" care has been uncovered (Ferrell, 2006). The nurses identified "aggressive care" and "aggressive care denying palliative care" as the most common conflicts causing distress. Their distress is the definition of their suffering and often comes through their identification with patient suffering. Table 4.3 includes examples from this survey regarding moral distress by oncology nurses.

Medical futility is defined as "care which is life sustaining and yet unlikely to result in meaningful survival" (Callahan, 2003). Another definition of futility is physiologic (Youngner 1988), where the intervention cannot be performed or is unlikely to be successful. This is the narrowest definition of futility and least value laden. The judgment is solely the physician's prerogative and is least whole-patient-centered. On the other hand, "qualitatively futile" (Schneiderman, Jecker, Jonsen, 1990) is highly value-laden, patient- and family-centered, and is consistent with Callahan's definition.

Conflict and feelings of moral distress occur when there is disagreement about futility of care between patient or family and the medical team or among the health-care team members. When there is conflict among the medical team about futility issues, nurses are often caught in the middle, trying to give the best possible care to the patient and support the families without becoming caught up in conflict.

Ethicists have recognized that participation in what is perceived as medically futile care creates moral distress in nurses and undermines the core of professional practice (Daly, 1994). In these situations, a nurse is the physician's agent, implementing medical directives of care. That role is highly conflicted when carrying out medical orders that the nurse believes will fail to do good and, in fact, may inflict further pain or harm.

Nurses are confronted with technological and pharmacological advances in all clinical settings. Means of respiratory and cardiac support, highly effective and yet also highly caustic antibiotics and chemotherapeutic agents, robotic surgeries, and organ transplantation provide the means to save the most critically ill and offer the miraculous reversal for what would otherwise be fatal problems (Callahan, 2003; Ahronheim, Morrison, Baskin, Morris, and Meier, 1996).

Tension develops from the technological ability to sustain life and the potential outcome of sustaining life beyond meaningful existence. A "successful" surgery, dialysis treatment, or resolved infection may represent a scientific achievement of goals at a cellular level but a disastrous outcome at a human level. Nurses are often left at the bedside of such "successes" as patients and their families are faced with the realities of prolonged life. Nurses also struggle with the public perception that the medical system can perform miracles, and nurses often report their own distress when witnessing patients and families agree to futile care offered by eager physicians and hospitals. Given the risk management concerns of health care, all providers

Table 4.3. Narratives of Moral Distress

My first experience with death, as a new nurse, was a frail man who came into the (ICU) after he coded at home. The patient coded again shortly after his arrival in the ICU. He was very frail, emaciated, and his body was a bright yellow-orange. The doctor in the unit was a young intern. He led the code. It was evident to all the nurses on the unit the code should not have been called. But the intern insisted on continuing. By the time he called off the code, there were many ribs broken. The memory of that patient has been etched in my mind since 1972.

72-year-old female with new diagnosis of lung cancer. Offered surgical excision of cancerous lung lobe. Pulmonary function tests prior to surgery indicated that respiratory function after surgery would probably be inadequate, requiring ventilation. Patient's husband insisted on surgery anyway, and patient was extubated 3 weeks after surgery. One day she was sitting up in a chair when she went into acute respiratory distress. At the bedside (I was a student nurse at the time), the patient grabbed my hand and pleaded, "Please let me go . . . Please just let me go." The medical residents arrived, reintubated the patient, inserted the nasogastric tube, which went into the patient's lungs and resulted in frothy bloody discharge from the mouth and nose. The patient remained sedated and ventilated in ICU another 2 weeks before dying.

I've been a nurse for 30 years, 25 of which have been focused on quality end-of-life care. I see more "suffering" today than I did 25 years ago. Our technology has surpassed our humanity, and our current focus on "technological brinkmanship" has increased cost while decreasing quality of life. As a nurse who has seen numerous "deaths" that occurred peacefully and gently, I am always saddened when I see one that isn't. I think it's extremely hard on nurses when all of our life experiences and lessons learned from these dying can't make an impact.

The patient had metastatic kidney cancer, sepsis, thrombocytopenia purpura, and was end-stage. But he was 58 years of age, a healthy man 6 months prior, and his wife was unable to let go, regardless of the knowledge presented to her with regard to the outcome. For 4 weeks, we kept this patient on dialysis, platelets, and red blood cells, transfused every other day. The patient was bleeding from the mouth; liver failure set in. He was looking like a corpse and his family was suffering every day. Yes, it was futile, expensive, and did not change the outcome. At the end his wife said, "Stop. It is not right transfusing all these blood products into my husband's dead body."

Mr. M was a 70-year-old man admitted for resection of a liver tumor. Post-op, he was admitted to our ICU. Mr. M had been in our ICU several weeks. He had never awakened post-op, and was ventilator-dependent. At the insistence of the nursing staff, we convened a multidisciplinary conference with the family. During the discussion, the physicians never used the words death or dying in spite of the fact that it was clear to them and the team that Mr. M would not survive hospitalization. It was clear that the family never completely understood the severity of the illness, so when they were asked to make decisions, they did not have the information to make an informed decision. I realized that as the nurse, I needed to function as not only the advocate, but also the interpreter.

A 72-year-old male patient had been admitted for scheduled colectomy for colon cancer. His post-op course involved multiple complications—bowel leak, peritonitis, infection, respiratory failure, renal failure, and skin breakdown, sepsis. The patient's family was adamant we continue all aggressive treatment per their religious beliefs. They could not withdraw support.

involved in twenty-first century health care—physicians, nurses, hospitals—err on the side of providing more care. "Defensive medicine" transcends to "defensive nursing," which often ultimately becomes patient suffering and shared suffering for all concerned.

Issues related to futile treatment have consistently been identified by nurses as among the most stressful aspects of critical care. Beckstrand and Kirchhoff (2005) conducted a survey that included responses from a national random sample involving 864 critical-care nurses. Among the most common obstacles to good end-of-life care, the most frequently reported by the nurses were disagreement about direction of dying patients' care; actions that prolonged patients' suffering; and physicians who were evasive and avoided conversations with family members. Other significant obstacles identified by the nurses included perceived family factors, such as lack of understanding about care, non-acceptance of poor prognoses, and overriding patients' advance directives.

Effective communication and mediation are key to resolving conflicts related to the goals of care. In 2003, Ahrens, Yancey, and Kollef reported results of a study of 43 patients who received care focused on facilitating family communication by a "communication team" of a physician and a nurse compared to 108 patients receiving usual care. Patients in the communication intervention group had shorter ICU stays, shorter hospital stays, and lower costs.

In 2001, a similar study involving 906 critical-care nurses was published. Of the nurses surveyed, Puntillo et al. reported that 34% indicated they sometimes had acted against their consciences, and 6% indicated they had done so to a great extent. In a similar study, Meltzer and Huckabay (2004) evaluated the relationship between nurses' perceptions of futile treatment and its effect on burnout. This study, which included 60 critical-care nurses, reported that nurses' emotional exhaustion was significantly related to the frequency of morally distressing situations regarding care perceived as futile or unbeneficial care.

In 2000, Ferrell, Virani, Grant, Coyne, and Uman conducted one of the few surveys on the topic of futile care and moral distress among oncology nurses. Data gathered from 2,333 nurses regarding end-of-life care reported common dilemmas such as discontinuing life-sustaining therapies and withholding or withdrawing nutrition or hydration. Family members' and health-care professionals' avoidance of the topic of death was cited as one of the barriers to effective care.

Three children's hospitals and four general hospitals with PICU were included in another survey. With a geographically diverse sample from the eastern, southwestern, and southern parts of the United States, the population-based sample was composed of attending physicians, house officers, and nurses who cared for children (ages 1 month to 18 years) with life-threatening conditions. All the patients were hospitalized in PICU or in medical, surgical, or hematology/oncology units. A total of 781 clinicians were sampled: 209 attending physicians, 116 house officers, and 456 nurses. About 54% of house officers and substantial proportions of attending physicians and nurses indicated that, "At times, I have acted against my conscience in providing treatment to children in my care." Of the different types of clinicians included in the study, 38% of critical-care attending physicians and 25% of hematology/oncology attending physicians expressed those concerns, whereas 48% of critical-care nurses and 38% of hematology/oncology nurses did so (Solomon et al., 2005).

An interesting finding is that nurses' own spirituality may influence their responses to suffering in a way similar to how patients and families facing the end of life confront their spirituality (Lo et al., 2003). One's faith may influence virtually all aspects of serious illness, including the meaning of life and death, the meaning of hope, and the ultimate power of God or a higher source (Nelson-Marten, Braaten and English, 2001). Nurses care for patients and families who may seek futile care based on a belief in miracles, and this may cause serious personal conflict. Nurses often support patients or families who believe God is the only worthy source of giving or ending life and whose health-care decisions reflect those beliefs. Indeed, nurses frequently struggle in an attempt to balance the patient and family's faith with their own and to balance personal and professional values.

Dorothee Soelle (1975), a scholar in political and liberation theology wrote *Suffering*, a text that discusses the mute suffering by a person who is stifled and reduced to silence when discourse is impossible. The sufferer becomes numb, speechless, and isolated. The person goes "inside himself" and loses the ability to act, think, or speak. He becomes submissive and feels powerless. Similarly, nurses may become silent when trapped between a demanding, unrealistic public and a health-care system willing to deliver futile care. This silencing may lead to a loss of personhood for the nurse and to stifling personal values and beliefs. The nurse may find it easier to become the automated, empty professional that Sulmasy (2006) warned was a possibility.

Soelle describes "lamenting" or "expressive suffering" as movement toward resolution. In the process, the person is able to analyze suffering's sources and to mobilize a response. In the final phase, those who have been oppressed feel solidarity and a sense of organization. They are then able to change structures that impose powerlessness.

In the survey cited earlier, the original version of the survey asked nurses to describe instances of moral distress they had experienced in witnessing medically futile care. In the first surveys collected, few nurses

Table 4.4. Examples of Religious or Spiritual Influences on Distress

I pray, "Please God, tell us when 'enough is enough.'" I thank God for colleagues and family who listen, support, and care. And it's by the grace of God that I am able to be strengthened each day, renewed each day, to do the Lord's work. Thank you for the opportunity to speak my heart's message.

We as humans do not have all the answers. As long as there is a will, there is life. How can anyone say this is hope? There can always be some benefit from our actions. Even if we can't see them.

The mother verbalized that she couldn't "give up and let her daughter die." We had offered chaplain support, but the family declined—I do believe that if she had allowed chaplain visits that she might have been more accepting of this death.

The patient was of the Catholic faith and had been active in her church family prior to a second stroke. The priest in the parish was older and felt that stopping dialysis was a form of suicide.

She was a faithful Southern Baptist, and her personal pastor told her she would "not go to heaven" if she stopped hemodialysis.

There is a time to end the "cure" phase and move onto the "care" phase. The outcome is not in our hands. When our work is finished, it's finished.

This patient had made a decision she wanted to die, and we should respect that. By trying to force a tube feeding on her, we were attacking her spirit. She had made her decision and her peace. It was disturbing to me that we were affecting her spirituality. I do not know what the next world will hold, the grave versus heaven versus limbo, waiting to come back. However, I believe that a peaceful death with family and friends and pets around would be more desired than the sounds of a ventilator, restrictions of restraints the glare of overhead light.

The staff required spiritual connection in this situation. They questioned, "Why, God, can I decide if this woman was to live or die?" They believed that they were administering lethal doses, and the responsibility of that hastening her death was fear. We focused daily on spiritual support for one another, the patient, and family. We had a prayer circle around the patient with staff, clergy, and the family.

I was angry with the medical staff for not taking responsibility for this man's suffering. I was confused and wanted the family to understand that sometimes God's miracle is heaven. I was fearful that this could easily have been me or one of my friends or family.

I kept asking God to take her. God tried, but the hospital staff wouldn't let go because of "policy."

My own personal spiritual beliefs of death with dignity were violated.

At this time, I did not invest much time in spirituality. Over the years, I have realized that the spiritual and religious factors play a huge role at the end of life.

My core value as a person and nurse is respect. I feel ashamed of the ways in which we violate patients.

I realized "hell was on earth" with what patients are put through. This made my being a patient advocate even stronger.

mentioned aspects of their own faith or spirituality. The survey was revised, and the subsequent participants in the survey were asked specifically to identify religious or spiritual factors that may have influenced their distress. The nurses completing this slightly revised survey provided rich narratives reflecting the influence of their spirituality in these circumstances. It is of tremendous interest that these intense feelings were not initially shared yet were clearly so much a part of the nurse's response to suffering. Table 4.4 includes examples from these responses.

SUMMARY

Nurses experience moral distress and suffering as well as rich rewards in their daily encounters with patients who are seriously ill or at the end of life. As frontline caregivers involved in intense and intimate care, nurses bear an enormous weight through feelings of responsibility from their cumulative experiences in caring for suffering patients. The observation described earlier—that nurses did not identify their own spirituality as a part of their professional work and experiences of suffering—warrants further investigation. The separation of mind, body, and spirit, which has been identified as a barrier to patient care, also prevails in professional education such that nurses may have been trained to distinguish their own faith and personhood from their role as nurses.

Nursing leaders in clinical practice settings and educators in both universities and continuing education can contribute much to the support of nurses through addressing the suffering of nurses.

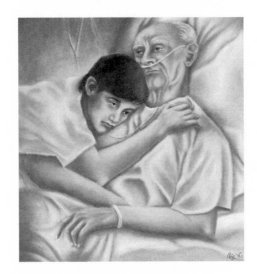

CHAPTER 5 ❦

What is the Nature of Suffering and What are the Goals of Nursing

In the earlier chapters we have explored the nature of suffering from the lens of nursing experience and through narratives of patients, family caregivers, and nurses themselves. We have also extracted essential themes from literature in nursing and other disciplines and through case examples that exemplify the structure of suffering.

Works by Eric Cassell and others in the field of medicine have informed our perspectives on suffering but, as we have argued, are not sufficient to describe the phenomenon of the suffering in the field of nursing. This is not surprising, as the nature of nursing is different from the nature of medicine. In addition, the power structure between medicine and nursing remains lopsided, perhaps influencing the experience of suffering for nurses. In reviewing both lay and professional literature, we are struck by how often the relief of suffering is attributed to the medical profession alone. We believe that this likely represents a broader paradigm in which the relief of suffering is meant to equal the cure of disease—a biomedical perspective that implies that the only true relief of suffering comes from fixing, curing, eliminating, and making free of illness, rather than the quality of a life lived. This paradigm should be rejected; it does not serve society well. But it may also reflect the "invisible" or "silent" aspect of nursing care that can have such a profound ameliorating effect on patient and family suffering.

Nurses play a fundamental role in caring for those who suffer. As a profession committed to the human response to illness or injury, the relief of suffering is at the core of nurses' work. Nurses are also dedicated to serving the most poor and vulnerable among us (Hughes, 2006). The care required may vary considerably, even among individuals with a similar diagnosis. Nothing is "routine" in caring for the seriously ill or dying. For example, the suffering of a person with AIDS may be dramatically different from one case to another. A middle-class African-American man with a dedicated partner and who lives in a comfortable environment with good access to health care is likely to experience a much different trajectory than the Caucasian homeless drug addict whose physiological experience of AIDS may be similar but whose life experience is not (Williams, 2004).

The previous chapters of this book have explored ethical and theological thought related to the nature of suffering. Nurses are intimately involved in whole-person care and, apart from the family, are the witnesses most often present as people in illness struggle with fundamental ethical concerns and spirituality. Emerging fields of thought, such as feminist ethics and humanities, have the opportunity to offer a broader paradigm beyond a single focus on cure. These perspectives also open the possibility that much suffering cannot be completely relieved, removed, or resolved but rather is witnessed, supported, accompanied, borne, and sometimes ameliorated through compassion and companionship. However, unnecessary suffering, as in that associated with pain and other symptoms, can almost always be relieved by expert care.

As a counter perspective to the issue of "Why God lets bad things happen to good people," Dr. Stanley Hauerwas, a Professor of Theological Ethics, wrote *Naming the Silences: God, Medicine, and the Problem of Suffering* (Hauerwas, 1990). This work instead asks why we seek answers to the "why?" question, using the context of dying children as an example of suffering and evil in the world. Hauerwas describes God as giving voice to our pain, and he names the silences created by unanswerable questions. He writes that modern medicine is a "noisy way to hide those silences" (Hauerwas, 1990, xi).

Theological questions about the problem of evil are central to exploring the nature of suffering. Hauerwas wrote:

> But sickness is quite another matter. Sickness should not exist because we think of it as something in which we can intervene and which we can ultimately eliminate. Sickness challenges our most cherished presumption that we are or at least can be in control of our existence. Sickness creates the problem of "anthropodicy" because it challenges our most precious and profound belief that

humanity has in fact become God. Against the backdrop of such a belief, we conclude that sickness should not exist. (Hauerwas, 1990, 62)

Suffering is thus viewed as an inherent part of illness because we, as people, have come to believe that the existence of untreatable illness is unjust and evil. Illness that cannot be cured is a threat to our integrity as humans because it informs us that we have no ultimate control—that illness and death will persist. In enduring illness, suffering can be transformative and provide meaning and ways of coping with chronic illness (Morse and Carter, 1996).

Hauerwas suggests that illness and suffering exist within a life story and that childhood suffering bothers us so intensely because we assume children do not yet have life stories to give their illness meaning. In the case of Christianity, he contends that Christians seek meaning and comfort in believing their lives are positioned in God's narrative (Hauerwas, 1990, 67). Hauerwas' contribution in *Naming the Silences* is that suffering exists within the context of stories, some "real" and others that are works of fiction. He concludes with a directive to caring people, whether professionals or lay companions, who observe suffering. He cites the story written by Nicholas Wolterstorff, *Lament for a Son*, who shares his grief:

> Death is awful, demonic. If you think your task as comforter is to tell me that really, all things considered, it's not so bad, you do not sit with me in my grief but place yourself off in the distance away from me. Over there, you are of no help. What I need to hear from you is that you recognize how painful it is. I need to hear from you that you are with me in my desperation. To comfort me, you have to come close. Come sit beside me on my mourning bench. (Hauerwas, 1990, 151)

Similar to the writing of Hauerwas, an important nursing contribution was made by Patricia Benner in her 1984 text *From Novice to Expert*. Benner described skill acquisition in nursing and the development of novice to expert nurses. Several examples of pain management and comfort are included in this work. The behaviors of expert nurses are described as committed and involved (Benner, 1984, 55–56) and contribute to the patient's sense of personhood, meaning, and dignity.

Benner suggests that the process of becoming an expert nurse creates confidence for nurses to know their "being" is as valuable—and in some cases more so—as their "doing." She also acknowledges that many nursing behaviors are not easily quantified. She concludes that "Nurses will not become more powerful or gain more status by ignoring their unique contributions simply because they are not easily replicated, standardized, or interpreted" (Benner, 1984, 75).

There are, however, some ways in which the roles of nursing and medicine overlap. Development of the roles of advanced nurse practitioners and clinical specialists, as well as increased acuity of care, have blurred many lines of responsibility. Yet there are significant aspects of care unique to nursing. One of these is the role of nurses in the intimate care of the body. The cleaning, touching, assessing, and attention to all the many devices that become connected to the hospitalized person requires a tremendous amount of bodily care by nurses. Bathing a patient, perhaps the most basic of nursing actions, affords an opportunity for intimate connection, private conversation, and comfort. Fagin and Diers wrote:

> Nursing is a metaphor for intimacy. Nurses are involved in the most private aspects of people's lives, and they cannot hide behind technology or a veil of omniscience as other practitioners or technicians in hospitals may do. Nurses do for others publicly what healthy persons do for themselves behind closed doors. Nurses, as trusted peers, are there to hear secrets, especially the ones born of vulnerability. Nurses are treasured when these interchanges are successful, but most often people do not wish to remember their vulnerability or loss of control, and nurses are indelibly identified with those terribly personal times. (Fagin and Diers, 1983, 116)

While many narratives about nurses are powerful depictions of unique circumstances, most are instead profound in their simplicity. Nurses' work actually resembles that of ordinary people enduring very stressful circumstances. A nurse in the fullest sense relates to suffering people with an authentic and gentle approach. A caring nurse offers calm to terrified parents in a NICU, assurance to the family awaiting the outcome of a surgery, hope to the patient receiving a first dose of chemotherapy, and consistent presence to the patient in long-term care.

While literature and the media often create a negative and inaccurate portrayal of nurses, there are some fictional portrayals of nurses that capture the essence of care. One such portrayal is found in *Range of Motion*, a novel by Elizabeth Berg. This is a story of Jay, a man who becomes comatose after being hit in the head by melting ice that falls from a building. Jay is transferred to a nursing home, and while most of his family and care providers have little hope for his recovery, his wife Lainey remains optimistic. She works continuously to maintain Jay's dignity while she waits, ever present, for his awakening.

One evening, Lainey returns to the nursing home and the nurse, Wanda, suggests that Lainey may want to lie down with Jay. The story continues:

'Just let me do something first,' Wanda says. She moves to the side of Jay's bed, pulls down the sheet. He is on his side, and she removes the pillow supporting him, holds him over with one hand while with the other she reaches for the bottle of lotion on his bedside stand. She's proud of the way Jay's skin has held up, no bedsores yet. She squirts some lotion into one hand, closes the bottle again and puts it back on the bedside stand. Nurses are good at this kind of thing, using one hand for things that normally require two. And if you get one like Wanda, you can see the caring along with the skill. She rubs Jay's back with strong, circular strokes, and I watch, spellbound. There is a mesmerizing quality to watching someone do almost anything with care: tailors in their dry-cleaner windows, hunched over sewing machines. Bakers making art out of frosting. Children with a new pack of crayons and fierce intent. We are meant to use what we have, whatever it is. We are meant to be less mindful of our insides, more outwardly directed. That's what I think, as I watch Wanda rub Jay down, as the minty smell of the lotion makes its way over to me. There is incredible value in being in service to others. (Berg, 1995).

This narrative aptly portrays the comforting care provided to the patient but also captures the effects on the observing family member.

Nurses can become, as Raphael (2003) described, "the face of God" to a patient and his family. Father Robert Smith, a Catholic priest, wrote of the ordinary in the profound nature of spiritual care:

As everyone knows, suffering appears in each human life, sometimes devastatingly; and its questions and challenges lie at the heart of every religious tradition. It can destroy lives and families, and it can deepen and transform them. The religious traditions contain centuries of hard-won wisdom, and their followers should become searchers within themselves, and companions for others, in the inescapable tests of human suffering. What is needed is not pious talk, but ordinary human courage, and the patient willingness to probe the mysteries of human and divine love. (Smith, 1996, 170)

Our exploration of the contextual analysis of suffering in Chapter 3 indicates that while the sources and contexts of suffering vary, the basic human responses are very similar. The source of "evil" may be a tumor, the unfairness of a baby born so prematurely that bodily organs can't sustain life, the unthinkable accident that leaves a young mother paralyzed, or the untimely occurrence of chronic diseases that may not result in bodily death but that dominate daily existence (Pinn, 1995). Beliefs in the nature of evil and how one interprets it under the circumstances of illness are reflected in ultimate issues of faith and spirituality (Penson et al., 2001).

Chapter 4 explored the contextual analysis of nurses' own suffering. To witness suffering in a close-up, bare, and intense way will likely result in our own personal pain. In the same way that the integrity of suffering patients and families is threatened, the integrity of nurses—individually and collectively as a profession—is threatened. The moral distress of nurses witnessing futile care is a model for the burden that goes alongside the rewards of our caring profession and the need for self-reflection, peer support, grieving, and, ultimately, to find meaning in our work and balance in our lives (Stairs, 2000).

As nurses, we are in an optimal position to share our stories, to be unafraid to speak of suffering, to learn from it, and to become proficient not only in the latest pharmacology or technology but also in our skills that will empower us to most effectively recognize and respond to suffering. Nurses who listen carefully and assess spiritual needs are able to understand what patients value most and what they hold sacred.

Schools of nursing and continuing education programs can teach the skills of listening, responding to anguish, hearing "why" questions, and in fundamentally re-envisioning what it means to be a nurse—perhaps even helping us return to our roots. We need these things soon, because as broken and burdened as our health-care system is, it is highly likely to get much worse before it gets better. The needs of an aging society, the demands of illness, the shortage of health-care professionals, and the global economy will each have a major impact.

There is cause for hope. Society has never needed nurses as much as they are needed today. Social changes, including the long overdue re-ordering of power structures and domination in society and in health care, have provided a space for the voice of nursing. Increasingly, yet certainly not sufficiently, the worlds of health care are recognizing that society's needs are best served by a multidisciplinary and interdisciplinary approach to care. The impact of complex cultural, psychological, and spiritual factors on health and well-being has also been acknowledged. Yet these aspects of care continue to be inadequately assessed and addressed.

FUNDAMENTAL TENETS OF THE NATURE OF SUFFERING AND THE GOALS OF NURSING

The literature in nursing, theology, ethics, psychology, and medicine collectively offer a deep understanding of suffering. Table 5.1 is a list we have

Table 5.1. Concepts Associated with Patient Suffering Derived from the Literature and Narratives

Abandoned	Injury	Pain
Affliction	Inner Distress	Powerlessness
Anguish	Isolation	Realization of What is Done/Not Done
Being Overwhelmed	Lacking a Voice	
Body Changes	Living in Apprehension	Resisting Loss
Brokenness	Living in Fear	Sadness
Coerced to do Treatment	Loneliness	Sense of Burden
Controlled by the Illness	Loss	Shared Experience
Depression	Loss of Control	Spiritual Pain
Deprivation	Loss of Dignity	Subjected to Violence
Despair	Loss of Everything That Once Was	Suffering is Experienced by Persons, not Bodies
Discomfort		
Emotional Pain	Loss of Self	Threat to the Wholeness of a Person
Enduring	Loss of Will to Live	
Evil	Lost Intimacy	To be Void of Meaning
Feeling Trapped	Multidimensional: Physical, Psycho, Social, Spiritual	To Hurt
Fighting to Live		To Lose Humor
Financial Distress	Mute Suffering	Trapped
Hair Loss	Needing Touch	Uncertainty
Helplessness	Not Accepting Death	Unrelieved, Relentless Pain
Hopelessness	Not Being Heard	Voice
Ignored/Feeling Diminished	Not Feeling at Peace	Vulnerability
	Not Relieved by Modern Medicine	Weary of Living
Immobilized		What Can't be put in Words but is Screaming to be Disclosed
Indescribable		
Individual Experience		

compiled of the descriptions of suffering synthesized from the literature cited in the previous chapters. In reviewing these key characteristics of suffering, the opportunities for nurses as well as the need for self-care become evident.

In reaching the synthesis across these chapters, we acknowledge the very significant earlier theoretical work of our nursing colleagues David Kahn and Richard Steeves (Kahn and Steeves, 1986, 1994, 1996). Their work, cited in Chapter 1, has provided a framework for nurses' understanding of suffering. Their scholarship laid the foundation for this book.

THE NATURE OF SUFFERING AND THE GOALS OF NURSING

What is the nature of suffering by patients and families enduring illness, and what are the goals of nursing in responding to these needs? While the latter question is not to be easily answered, we conclude with an attempt to provide an initial schema of tenets that respond to this question. It is our hope that these tenets will provide some insight previously unavailable to nurses and will also open doors to further reflection and scholarship. Many of these tenets apply to the suffering of nurses as well as those they care for. The tenets are:

1. Suffering is described as a loss of control, which creates insecurity. Suffering people often feel helpless and trapped, unable to escape their circumstances.
2. In most instances, suffering is associated with loss. The loss may be of a relationship or of some aspect of the self, or loss of some aspect of the physical body. The loss may be evident only in the mind of the sufferer, but it nonetheless leaves a person feeling diminished and with a sense of brokenness.
3. Suffering is an intensely personal experience.
4. Suffering is accompanied by a range of intense emotions including sadness, anguish, fear, abandonment, despair, and a myriad of other emotions.
5. Suffering can be deeply linked to a recognition of one's own mortality. When threatened by serious illness, people may fear the end of life. Conversely, for others, living with serious illness may cause a yearning for death.
6. Suffering often involves asking the question "Why?" Illness or loss my be seen as untimely and undeserved. Suffering people seek to find meaning and answers for that which is unknowable.
7. Suffering is often associated with separation from the world. Individuals may express intense loneliness and yearn for connection with others while also feeling intense distress about dependency on others.
8. Suffering is often accompanied by spiritual distress. Regardless of religious affiliation, individuals experiencing illness may feel a sense of hopelessness. When life is threatened, there may be a self-evaluation of what has been lived and what remains undone. Becoming weak and vulnerable and

facing mortality may cause one to reevaluate his/her relationship with a higher being.

9. Suffering is not synonymous with pain but is closely associated with it. Physical pain is closely related to psychological, social, and spiritual distress. Pain which persists without meaning becomes suffering.

10. Suffering occurs when the individual feels voiceless. This may occur when the person is mute to give words to their experience or when their "screams" are unheard.

Nurses are the confidants for patients who experience the personal threat of injury or serious illness. Through their provision of competent care for pain and other symptoms and through their relief of physical problems, nurses can reduce the psychological, social, and spiritual distress of the person. The intimate care of the physical body offers nurses a special opportunity for healing brokenness and helping to restore a sense of dignity and worth. Nurses recognize that witnessing suffering is a part of their daily work, yet they seek to understand each person who is suffering as a unique individual. Nurses respond to suffering first and foremost through *presence*. As witnesses to suffering, they serve as a compassionate voice that recognizes the human response to illness amidst the chaos and depersonalization of the health-care environment.

The writing of physician Rachel Naomi Remen speaks to the work of nursing as a service to others. Remen writes of the distinction between helping versus serving others. She says that "serving is different from helping in that helping is based on inequality; it is not a relationship between equals. Serving is a relationship between equals" (Remen 1996). Remen writes:

There is distance between ourselves and whatever or whomever we are fixing. Fixing is a form of judgment. All judgment creates distance, a disconnection, an experience of difference. In fixing there is an inequality of expertise that can easily become a moral distance. We cannot serve at a distance. We can serve only that to which we are profoundly connected, that which we are willing to touch. This is Mother Teresa's basic message. We serve life not because it is broken but because it is holy. (Remen, 1996, 24)

Remen also writes of how serving sustains us as health-care providers. She says that "our service serves us as well as others. That which uses us strengthens us. Over time, fixing and helping are draining, depleting. Over time we burn out. Service is renewing. When we serve, our work itself will sustain us" (Remen, 1996, 24).

Through listening to their patients, nurses can help the person move beyond mute suffering to expressing their emotional distress. This distress often includes expression of sadness, loneliness, fear, helplessness, hopelessness, and a sense of brokenness. Nurses can ameliorate distress and help restore wholeness through this human connection. They respond to the spiritual distress of suffering, regardless of the suffering person's religious affiliation. To do this, nurses are called on to reflect on their own spirituality.

Helping patients regain control in the face of illness and to cope with the vulnerability and uncertainty of life is part of nursing care. The nurse accompanies patients on their journey, and through this ongoing and intimate encounter they support the patient in confronting the weariness of living and dying as well as the struggle for life. As witnesses, nurses support patients who seek meaning from their distressing circumstances. Through the intimacy of caring, nurses also experience personal suffering and respond by seeking a balance of life and work and through deep personal reflection. This is the challenging and rewarding work of nursing.

References

Agency for Health Care Policy and Research. (1994). *Clinical practice guideline cancer pain management*. Rockville, MD: United States Department of Health and Human Services.

Agnus, D.C., A.E. Barnato, W.T. Linde-Zwirbler, L.A. Weissfeld, R.S. Walson, and T. Ricket, et al. (2004). Use of intensive care at the end of life in the United States: an epidemiologic study. *Critical Care Medicine*, 32: 638–643.

American Cancer Society. (2006). Facts and Figures. Atlanta: American Cancer Society.

Ahrens, T., V. Yancey, and M. Kollef. (2003). Improving family communications at the end of life: Implications for length of stay in the intensive care unit and resource use. *American Journal of Critical Care*, 12: 317–323.

Ahronheim, J.C., R.S. Morrison, S.A. Baskin, J. Morris, and D.E. Meier. (1996). Treatment of the dying in the acute care hospital. Advanced dementia and metastatic cancer. *Archives of Internal Medicine*, 156: 2094–2100.

Alken, M. (1997). *The healing power of forgiving*. New York: Crossroad Publishing Company.

Arman, M., A. Rehnsfeldt, L. Lindholm, and E. Hamrin. (2002). The face of suffering among women with breast cancer. *Cancer Nursing*, 25: 96–103.

Ashby, H.U. (2003). Being forgiven: toward a thicker description of forgiveness. *The Journal of Pastoral Care and Counseling*, 57: 143–152.

Baines, B.K., and L. Norlander. (2000). The relationship of pain and suffering in a hospice population. *American Journal of Hospice and Palliative Care*, 17: 319–326.

Battenfield, B.L. (1984). Suffering: A conceptual description and content analysis of operational schema. *Journal of Nursing Scholarship*, 16: 36–41.

Beckstrand, R.L., and K.T. Kirchhoff. (2005). Providing end-of-life care to patients: Critical care nurses' perceived obstacles and supportive behaviors. *American Journal of Critical Care*, 14: 395–403.

Benedict, S. (1989). The suffering associated with lung cancer. *Cancer Nursing*, 12: 34–40.

Benner, P. (1984). *From Novice to Expert*. Redwood City, CA: Addison Wesley Publishing Company.

Benner, P., S. Kerchner, I.B. Corless, and B. Davies. (2003). Attending death as a human passage: core nursing principles for end of life care. *American Journal of Critical Care*, 12: 558–561.

Berg, E. (1995). *Range of Motion*. New York: Berkley Books.

Berry, P., and J. Griffe. (2006). Planning for the actual death. In B. R. Ferrell and N. Coyle *(Eds.)*, *Textbook of Palliative Nursing*, pp. 561–577. New York: Oxford University Press.

Bershady, H. (1992). *Max Scheler. On Feeling, Knowing, and Valuing*. Chicago: University of Chicago Press.

Boland, D., and S. Sims. (1996). Family caregiving at home as a solitary journey. *Image: Journal of Nursing Scholarship*, 28: 55–58.

Borneman, T., and K. Brown-Saltzman. (2006). Meaning in illness. In B.R. Ferrell and N. Coyle *(Eds.)*, *Textbook of Palliative Nursing*, pp. 605–616. New York: Oxford University Press.

Borneman, T., D.Z.J. Chu, L. Wagman, B. Ferrell, G. Juarez, L E. McCahill, and G. Uman. (2003). Concerns of family caregivers of patients with cancer facing palliative surgery for advanced malignancies. *Oncology Nursing Forum*, 30: 997–1005.

Breitbart, W. (2002). Spirituality and meaning in supportive care. Spirituality and meaning-centered group psychotherapy interventions in advanced cancer. *Supportive Care in Cancer*, 10: 272–280.

Callahan, D. (2003). Living and dying with medical technology. *Critical Care Medicine*, 31 (Suppl. 5): S344–S346.

Cannon, K. (1995). *Katie's Canon. Womanism and the soul of the black community*. New York: Continuum.

Cassell, E.J. (1999). Diagnosing suffering: A perspective. *Annals of Internal Medicine*, 131: 531–534.

———. (1991). *The Nature of Suffering and the Goals of Medicine*. Oxford: Oxford University Press.

———. (1982). The Nature of Suffering and the Goals of Medicine. *New England Journal of Medicine*, 306: 639–645.

Chapman, C.R., and I. Gavrin. (1999). Suffering: The contributions of persistent pain. *The Lancet*, 353: 2233–2237.

Charmaz, K. (1983). Loss of self: A fundamental form of suffering in the chronically ill. *Sociology of Health & Illness*, 5: 168–195.

Cherny, N.I, N. Coyle, and K.M. Foley. (1994). Suffering in the advanced cancer patient: A definition and taxonomy. *Journal of Palliative Care*, 10: 57–70.

Chiu, L. (2000). Transcending breast cancer, transcending death: A Taiwanese population. *Nursing Science Quarterly*, 13: 64–72.

Chochinov, H.M. (2006). Dying, dignity, and new horizons in palliative end-of-life care. *CA: A Cancer Journal for Clinicians*, 56: 84–103.

Chochinov, H.M., T. Hack, T. Hassard, L.J. Kristjanson, S. McClement, and M. Harlos. (2002). Dignity in the terminally ill: A cross-sectional cohort study. *The Lancet*, 360: 2026–2030.

Cohen, M.A., and B. Sarter. (1992). Love and work: Oncology nurses' view of the meaning of their work. *Oncology Nursing Forum*, 19: 1481–1486.

Collins, C., M. Liken, S. King, and C. Kokinakis. (1993). Loss and grief among family caregivers of relatives with dementia. *Qualitative Health Research*, 3: 236–253.

Copp, L.A. (1974). The spectrum of suffering. *American Journal of Nursing*, 74: 491–494.

———. (1990a). The nature and prevention of suffering. *Journal of Professional Nursing*, 6: 247–249.

———. (1990b). Treatment, torture, suffering, and compassion. *Journal of Professional Nursing*, 6: 1–2.

Coyle, N. (2006). The hard work of living in the face of death. *Journal of Pain and Symptom Management*, 32: 266–274.

———. (2004). The "existential slap:" A crisis of disclosure. *International Journal of Palliative Nursing,* 10: 520.

———. (1996). Suffering in the first person: Glimpses of suffering through patients' and family narratives. In B.R. Ferrell *(Ed.)*, *Suffering*, pp. 29–64. Sudbury, MA: Jones & Bartlett.

Dahlin, C., and D. Giansiracusa. (2006). Communication in palliative care. In B. R. Ferrell and N. Coyle *(Eds.)*, *Textbook of Palliative Nursing*, pp. 67–93. New York: Oxford University Press.

Daly, B.J. (1994). Futility. *AACN Clinical Issues in Critical Care Nursing*, 5: 77–85.

Daneault, S., V. Lussier, S. Mongeau, P. Paille, E. Hudon, D. Dion, et al. 2004. The nature of suffering and its relief in the terminally ill. *Journal of Palliative Care*, 20: 7–11.

Davies, B. (2006). Supporting families in palliative care. In B. R. Ferrell and N. Coyle *(Eds.)*, *Textbook of Palliative Nursing*, pp. 545–560. New York: Oxford University Press.

Desbians, N.A., and A. Wu. (2000). Pain and suffering in seriously ill hospitalized patients. *Journal of the American Geriatrics Society*, 48(5 Suppl): S183–S186.

Dow, K.H., B.R. Ferrell, M.R. Haberman, and L. Eaton. (1999). The meaning of quality of life in cancer survivorship. *Oncology Nursing Forum*, 26: 519–528

Duggleby, W. (2000). Enduring suffering: A grounded theory analysis of the pain experience of elderly hospice patients with cancer. *Oncology Nursing Forum*, 27: 825–831.

Enright, R.D., and C.T. Coyle. (1998). Researching the process model of forgiveness within psychological interventions. In E.L. Worthington *(Ed.)*, *Dimensions of Forgiveness: Psychological Research and Theological Perspectives*, pp. 139–161. Philadelphia, PA: Templeton Foundation Press.

Ersek, M. (2006). The meaning of hope in the dying. In B.R. Ferrell and N. Coyle *(Eds.)*, *Textbook of Palliative Nursing*, pp. 513–529. New York: Oxford University Press.

Ersek, M., and S.A. Wilson. (2003). The challenges and opportunities in providing end-of-life care in nursing homes. *Journal of Palliative Medicine*, 6: 45–57.

Ersek, M., and B.R. Ferrell. (1994). Providing relief from cancer pain by assisting in the search for meaning. *Journal of Palliative Care*, 10: 15–22.

Ersek, M., B.R. Ferrell, and K. H. Dow, and C. H. Melancon. (1997). Quality of life in women with ovarian cancer. *Western Journal of Nursing Research*, 19: 334–350.

Fagin, C., and D. Diers. (1983). Nursing as metaphor: Occasional notes. *New England Journal of Medicine*, 309: 116.

Fall-Dickson, J.M., and L. Rose. (1999). Caring for patients who experience chemotherapy-induced side effects: The meaning for oncology nurses. *Oncology Nursing Forum*, 26: 901–907.

Farley, M. (2002). *Compassionate Respect: A Feminist Approach to Medical Ethics and Other Questions*. Mahwah, NJ: Paulist Press.

Farley, W. (1990). *Tragic Vision and Divine Compassion: A Contemporary Theodicy*. Louisville, KY: Westminster John Knox Press.

Ferrell, B.R. (2006). Understanding the moral distress of nurses witnessing medically futile care. *Oncology Nursing Forum*, 33: 922–930.

———. (2005). Ethical perspectives on pain and suffering. *Pain Management Nursing*, 6: 83–90.

———. (2001). Pain observed: The experience of pain from the family caregiver's perspective. *Clinics in Geriatric Medicine*, 3: 595–609.

———. (1996). The quality of lives: 1,525 voices of cancer. *Oncology Nursing Forum*, 23: 907–916.

———. (1993). To know suffering. *Oncology Nursing Forum*, 20: 1471–1477.

Ferrell, B.R., and V. Sun. (2006). Suffering. In R. M. Carroll-Johnson, L. M. Gorman, and N. J. Bush *(Eds.)*, *Psychosocial Nursing Care Along the Cancer Continuum*, pp. 155–168. Pittsburgh, PA: ONS Publishing Division.

Ferrell, B.R., S.L. Smith, G. Juarez, and C. Melancon. (2003). Meaning of illness and spirituality in ovarian cancer survivors. *Oncology Nursing Forum*, 30: 249–257.

Ferrell, B.R., K. Ervin, S. Smith, T. Marek, and C. Melancon. (2002). Family perspectives of ovarian cancer. *Cancer Practice*, 10: 269–276.

Ferrell, B.R, R. Virani, M. Grant, P. Coyne, and G. Uman. (2000). Beyond the Supreme Court decision: Nursing perspectives on end-of-life care. *Oncology Nursing Forum*, 27: 445–455.

Ferrell, B.R., M. Grant, and R. Virani. (1999). Strengthening nursing education to improve end-of-life care. *Nursing Outlook*, 47: 252–256.

Ferrell B.R., R. Virani, and M.M. Grant. (1999). Analysis of end-of-life content in nursing textbooks. *Oncology Nursing Forum*, 26: 869–876.

Ferrell, B.R., M.M. Grant, B. Funk, S. Otis-Green, and N. Garcia. (1997). Quality of life in breast cancer survivors as identified by focus groups. *Pyscho-Oncology*, 6: 13–23.

Ferrell, B.R., M. Grant, G.E. Dean, B. Funk, and J. Ly. (1996). "Bone Tired": The Experience of Fatigue and Its Impact on Quality of Life. *Oncology Nursing Forum*, 23: 1539–1547.

Ferrell, B.R., K.H. Dow, S. Leigh, J. Ly, and P. Gulasekaram. (1995). Quality of life in long-term cancer survivors. *Oncology Nursing Forum*, 22: 915–922.

Ferrell, B.R., M. Rhiner, B. Shapiro, and M. Dierkes. (1994). The experience of pediatric cancer pain. Part I: Impact of pain on the family. *Journal of Pediatric Nursing*, 9: 368–379.

Ferrell, B.R., E.J. Taylor, G. R. Sattler, M. Fowler, and B. L. Cheyney. (1993). Searching for the meaning of pain: Cancer patients,' caregivers,' and nurses' perspectives. *Cancer Practice*, 1: 185–194.

Ferrell, B.R., M. Rhiner, M.Z. Cohen, and M. Grant. (1991). Pain as a metaphor for illness part I: Impact of cancer pain on family caregivers. *Oncology Nursing Forum*, 18: 1303–1309.

Fox, M. (2001). *Prayer: A Radical Perspective*. New York: Penguin Putnam, Inc.

Frankl, V. (1963). *Man's Search for Meaning: An Introduction to Logotherapy*. New York: Pocket Books.

Ganzini, L., W.S. Johnston, and W.F. Hoffman. (1999). Correlates of suffering in amyotrophic lateral sclerosis. *Neurology*, 52: 1434–1440.

Gilligan, C. (1982). *In a Different Voice*. Cambridge, MA: Harvard University Press.

Grant, M., B.R. Ferrell, G.M. Schmidt, P. Fonbuena, J.C. Niland, and S.J. Forman. (1992). Measurement of quality of life in bone marrow transplant survivors. *Quality of Life Research*, 1: 375–384.

Greipp, M. (1992). Undermedication for pain: An ethical model. *Advances in Nursing Science*, 15: 44–53.

Harper, B. (1994). *Death: The Coping Mechanism of the Health Professional*. Greenville, SC: Southeastern University Press.

Harrison, B.W. (1985). *Making the Connections: Essays in Feminist Social Ethics*. Boston: Beacon Press.

Hauerwas, S. (1990). *Naming the Silences: God, Medicine, and the Problem of Suffering*. London: T & T Clark International.

Held, V. (Ed.) (1995). *Justice and Care: Essential Readings in Feminist Ethics*. Boulder, CO: Westview Press.

Heschel, A. (1955). *God in Search of Man: A Philosophy of Judaism*. New York: Farrar, Straus and Giroux.

Hickman, S.E., V.P. Tilden, and S. W. Tolle. (2004). Family perceptions of worry, symptoms, and suffering in the dying. *Journal of Palliative Care*, 20: 20–27.

Hill, C.S. (1992). Suffering as contrasted to pain, loss, grief, despair, and loneliness. In P. Starck and J. McGovern *(Eds.)*, *The Hidden Dimension of Illness: Human Suffering*, pp. 69–80. New York: National League for Nursing.

Hoffman, D.E., and A.J. Tarzian. (2001). The girl who cried pain: A bias against women in the treatment of pain. *Journal of Law, Medicine, and Ethics*, 29: 13–27.

Horowitz, K.E., and D.M. Lanes. (1992). *Witness to Illness: Strategies for Caregiving and Coping.* Reading, MA: Addison-Wesley.

Hughes, A. (2006). Poor, homeless, and underserved populations. In B.R. Ferrell and N. Coyle *(Eds.), Textbook of Palliative Nursing*, pp. 661–670. New York: Oxford University Press.

Institute of Medicine. (2005). *From Cancer Patient to Cancer Survivor: Lost in Transition.* Washington D.C.: National Academies Press.

———. (2002). *When Children Die: Improving Palliative and End-of-Life Care for Children and Their Families.* Washington D.C.: National Academies Press.

Jackson, K. (2003). *The Gift to Listen, the Courage to Hear.* Minneapolis: Augsburg Fortress Publishers.

Jaggar, A.M. (1989). Love and knowledge: Emotion in feminist epistemology. In A. Garry and M. Pearsall *(Eds.), Women, Knowledge, and Reality.* Boston: Unwin Hyman.

Juarez, G., B. Ferrell, and T. Borneman. (1998). Perceptions of quality of life in Hispanic patients with cancer. *Cancer Practice*, 6: 318–324.

Kagawa-Singer, M. (1994). Diverse cultural beliefs and practices about death and dying in the elderly. In D. Wieland, D. Benton, and B. Kramer, *(Eds.), Cultural Diversity and Geriatrics Care: Challenges to the Health Professions*, pp. 101–116. Binghamton, NY: Hayworth Press.

Kahn, D.L., and R.H. Steeves. (1996). An understanding of suffering grounded in clinical practice and research. In B.R. Ferrell *(Ed.), Suffering*, pp. 3–28. Sudbury, MA: Jones & Bartlett.

———. (1994). Witnesses to suffering: Nursing knowledge, voice, and vision. *Nursing Outlook*, 42: 260–264.

———. (1986). The experience of suffering: Conceptual clarification and theoretical definition. *Journal of Advanced Nursing*, 11: 623–631.

Kemp, C. (2006). Spiritual care interventions. In B.R. Ferrell and N. Coyle *(Eds.), Textbook of Palliative Nursing*, pp. 595–604. New York: Oxford University Press.

Kirchhoff, K.T., R.L. Beckstrand, and P.R. Anamandla. (2003). Analysis of end-of-life content in critical care nursing textbooks. *Journal of Professional Nursing*, 19: 372–381.

Kirchhoff K.T., Song, M.K., and Kehl, K. (2004). Caring for the family of the critically ill patient. Critical Care Clinics 20: 453–66.

Kleinman, A. (1988). *The Illness Narratives.* New York: Basic Books.

Kumasaka, L., and A. Miles. (1996). My pain is God's will. *American Journal of Nursing*, 96: 45–47.

Kuuppalomaki, M., and L. Sirkka. (1998). Cancer patients' reported experiences of suffering. *Cancer Nursing*, 21: 364–369.

Lartey, E.Y. (2003). *In Living Color: An Intercultural Approach to Pastoral Care and Counseling.* 2nd Ed. London: Jessica Kingsley Publishers.

Lederberg, M. (1998). The family of the cancer patient. In J. Holland *(Ed.)*, *Psycho-Oncology*. New York: Oxford University Press.

Lewis, F.M., and L.W. Deal. (1995). Balancing our lives: A study of the married couples' experience with breast cancer recurrence. *Oncology Nursing Forum*, 22: 943–953.

Lin, H.R. and S.M. Bauer-Wu. (2003). Psycho-spiritual well-being in patients with advanced cancer: An integrative review of the literature. *Journal of Advanced Nursing*, 44: 69–80.

Lo, B., L. W. Kates, D. Ruston, R.M. Arnold, C.B. Cohen, C.M. Puchalski, et al. (2003). Responding to requests regarding prayer and religious ceremonies by patients near the end of life and their families. *Journal of Palliative Medicine*, 6: 409–415.

Loeser, J.D. (2000). Pain and suffering. *Clinical Journal of Pain*, 16(2 suppl): S2–S6. *Cancer Nursing*, 29: 120–131.

Madjar, I. (1998). *Giving Comfort and Inflicting Pain*. Edmonton, Alberta, Canada: Qual Institute Press.

Madjar, I. and J.A. Walton *(Eds.)* (1999). *Nursing and the Experience of Illness*. London: Routledge.

Mazanec, P. (2007). *Distant Caregiving for a Parent with Advanced Cancer*. Unpublished doctoral dissertation. Case Western Reserve University: Frances Payne Bolton School of Nursing.

McCaffery, M. (1968). *Nursing practice theories related to cognition, bodily pain, and main environment interactions*. Los Angeles: University of California Los Angeles.

McClain-Jacobsen, C., B. Rosenfeld, A. Kosinski, H. Pessin, J.E. Cimino, and W. Breitbart (2004). Belief in afterlife, spiritual well-being and end-of-life despair in patients with advanced cancer. *General Hospital Psychiatry*, 26: 484–486.

McCullough, M., K.I. Pargament, and C.E. Thoreson *(Eds.)* (2000). *Forgiveness: Theory, Research, and Practice*. New York: The Guilford Press.

McGrath, P. (2002). Creating a language for spiritual pain through research: A beginning. *Supportive Care in Cancer*, 10: 637–646.

Meinhart, N., and M. McCaffery. (1990). *Pain: A Nursing Approach to Assessment and Analysis*. Norwalk, CT: Appleton-Century-Crofts.

Meltzer, L.S., and L.M. Huckabay. (2004). Critical care nurses' perceptions of futile care and its effect on burnout. *American Journal of Critical Care*, 13: 202–208.

Miaskowski, C., E.F. Zimmer, K.M. Barrett, S.L. Dibble, and M. Wallhagen. (1997). Differences in patients' and family caregivers' perceptions of the pain experience influence patient and caregiver outcomes. *Pain*, 72: 217–226.

Morse, J.M., and B. Carter. (1996). The essence of enduring and expressions of suffering: The reformulation of self. *Scholarly Inquiry for Nursing Practice*, 10: 43–60.

Morse, S.T., and B. Fife. (1998). Coping with a partner's cancer: adjustment at four stages of the illness trajectory. *Oncology Nursing Forum*, 25: 751–760.

Mullan, F. (1985). Seasons of survival: Reflections of a physician with cancer. *New England Journal of Medicine*, 313: 270–273.

Muller-Fahrenholz, G. (1997). *The Art of Forgiveness: Theological Reflections on Healing and Reconciliation*. Geneva: WCC Publications.

Nelson, J.E., D.E. Meier, E.J. Oei, D.M. Nierman, R.S. Senzel, P.L. Manfredi, et al. (2001). Self-reported symptom experience of critically ill cancer patients receiving intensive care. *Critical Care Medicine*, 29: 277–282.

Nelson-Marten, P., J. Braaten, and N.K. English. (2001). Critical caring. Promoting good end-of-life care in the intensive care unit. *Critical Care Nursing Clinics of North America*, 13: 577–585.

Northouse, L.L., D. Mood, T. Kershaw, A. Schafenacker, S. Mellon, J. Walker, et al. (2002). Quality of life of women with recurrent breast cancer and their family members. *Journal of Clinical Oncology*, 20: 4050–4064.

Nouwen, H.J.M. (1991). *The Way of the Heart: Desert Spirituality and Contemporary Ministry*. San Francisco, CA: Harper San Francisco.

O'Connor, K.F. (1996). Ethical/moral experiences of oncology nurses. *Oncology Nursing Forum*, 23: 787–794.

O'Connor, A., C. Wicker, and B. Germino. (1990). Understanding the cancer patient's search for meaning. *Cancer Nursing*, 13: 167–175.

Pasacreta, J.V., P.A. Minarik, and L. Nield-Anderson. (2006). Anxiety and depression. In B.R. Ferrell and N. Coyle *(Eds.)*, *Textbook of Palliative Nursing*, pp. 375–399. New York: Oxford University Press.

Pinn, A. (1995). *Why Lord? Suffering and Evil in Black Theology*. New York: Continuum.

Penson, R.T., R.Z. Yusuf, B.A. Chabner, J.P. LaFrancesca, M. McElhinny, A.S. Axelrad, et al. (2001). Losing God. *The Oncologist*, 6: 286–297.

Potter, M. (2006). Loss, suffering bereavement and grief. In M.L. Matzo and D.W. Sherman *(Eds.)*, *Palliative Care Nursing: Quality Care to the End of Life*, pp. 273–315. New York: Springer Publishing Company.

Prendergast, T.J. and J.M. Luce. (1997). Increasing incidence of withholding and withdrawal of life support from the critically ill. *American Journal of Respiratory and Critical Care Medicine*, 155: 15–20.

Price, B. (1996). Illness careers: The chronic illness experience. *Journal of Advanced Nursing*, 24: 275–279.

Prince-Paul, M. (2006). *Relationships Among Communicative Acts, Social Well-Being, and Spirituality on the Quality of Life at the End of Life*. Unpublished doctoral dissertation. Case Western Reserve University: Frances Payne Bolton School of Nursing.

Proctor-Smith, M. (1995). *Praying with Our Eyes Open: Engendering Feminist Liturgical Power*. Nashville, TN: Abingdon Press.

Puchalski, C.M., Rabbi E. Dorff, and I.Y. Hendi. (2004). Spirituality, religion, and healing in palliative care. *Clinics in Geriatric Medicine*, 20: 689–714.

Puntillo, K.A., P. Benner, T. Drought, B. Drew, N. Stotts, D. Stannard, et al. (2001). End-of-life issues in intensive care units: A national random survey of nurses; knowledge and beliefs. *American Journal of Critical Care*, 10: 216–229.

Raphael, M. (2003). *The Female Face of God in Auschwitz.* New York: Routledge Press.

Reich, W.T. (1989). Speaking of suffering: A moral account of compassion. *Soundings,* 72: 83–108.

———. (1987). Models of pain and suffering: Foundations for an ethic of compassion. *Acta Neurochirurgica Supplementum,* 38: 117–122.

Remen, R.N. (1996). In the service of life. *Noetic Sciences Review,* 37: 24–26.

Rodgers, B.L., and K.V. Cowles. (1997). A conceptual foundation for human suffering in nursing care and research. *Journal of Advanced Nursing,* 25: 1048–1053.

Sachs, G.A. (1988). On deeper reflection. *Journal of the American Medical Association,* 259: 2145.

Scarry, E. (1985). *The Body in Pain.* New York: Oxford University Press.

Scheler, M. (1962). *Man's Place in Nature.* Translated by H. Meyerhoff. New York: Farrar Straus and Cudahy.

Schneiderman, L.J., N. S. Jecker, and A.R. Jonsen. (1990) Medical futility: its meaning and ethical implications. *Annals of Internal Medicine,* 112: 949–54.

Shannon, S. (2001). Helping families cope with death in the ICU. In J.R. Curtis and G. Rubenfeld *(Eds.), Managing Death in the Intensive Care Unit—The Transition from Cure to Comfort,* pp. 165–182. New York: Oxford University Press.

Shapiro, B.S. (1996). The suffering of children and their families. In B. R. Ferrell *(Ed.), Suffering,* pp. 67–94. Sudbury, MA: Jones & Bartlett.

Sherman, S.E., and D. Reuben. (1998). Measures of functional status in community-dwelling elders. *Journal of General Internal Medicine,* 13: 817–823.

Smith, R. (1996). Theological perspectives. In B.R. Ferrell *(Ed.), Suffering,* pp. 159–172. Sudbury, MA: Jones & Bartlett.

Soelle, D. (1975). *Suffering.* Philadelphia: Fortress Press.

Solomon, M.Z., D.E. Sellers, K.S. Heller, D.L. Dokken, M. Levetown, C. Rushton, et al. (2005). New and lingering controversies in pediatric end-of-life care. *Pediatrics,* 116: 872–883.

Springstead, E.O. (1998). *Simone Weil.* Maryknoll, NY: Orbis Books.

Spross, J. A. (1996). Coaching and suffering: The role of the nurse in helping people facing illness. In B.R. Ferrell *(Ed.), Suffering,* pp. 173–208. Sudbury, MA: Jones & Bartlett.

Stairs, J. (2000). *Listening for the Soul: Pastoral Care and Spiritual Direction.* Minneapolis: Augsburg Fortress Publishers.

Stanley, K.J., and L. Zoloth-Dorfman. (2006). Ethical considerations. In B.R. Ferrell and N. Coyle *(Eds.), Textbook of Palliative Nursing,* pp. 1031–1052. New York: Oxford University Press.

Stark, P.L., and J.P. McGovern. (1992). The meaning of suffering. In P.L. Stark, and J.P. McGovern *(Eds.), The Hidden Dimension of Illness: Human Suffering,* pp. 25–42. New York: National League for Nursing Press.

Steeves, R.H. (1988). *The Experiences of Suffering and Meaning in Bone Marrow Transplant Patients.* Unpublished doctoral dissertation. Seattle, WA: University of Washington.

Steeves, R.H., M.Z. Cohen, and C.T. Wise. (1994). An analysis of critical incidents describing the essence of oncology nursing. *Oncology Nursing Forum*, 21 (Suppl. 8): 19–25.

Sulmasy, D.P. (2006). *The Rebirth of the Clinic: An Introduction to Spirituality in Health Care*. Washington, D.C.: Georgetown University Press.

Talerico, K.A. (2003). Grief and older adults. Differences, issues, and clinical approaches. *Journal of Psychosocial Nursing and Mental Health Services*, 41: 12–16.

Taylor, C.R. and R. Dell'Oro *(Eds.)*. (2006). *Health and Human Flourishing*. Washington, D.C.: Georgetown University Press.

Tong, R. (1993). *Feminine and Feminist Ethics*. Belmont, CA: Wadsworth Press.

Townes, E. (1995). *In a Blaze of Glory*. Nashville: Abingdon Press.

Travelbee, J. (1971). Illness and suffering as human experiences. In *Interpersonal aspects of Nursing*, pp. 86–89. Philadelphia: F. A. Davis Company.

Walton, J.A. (1999). On living with schizophrenia. In I. Madjar and J.A. Walton *(Eds.)*, *Nursing and the Experience of Illness. Phenomenology in Practice*, pp. 98–122. London: Routledge.

Weatherhead, L.D. (1936). *Why do Men Suffer?* Nashville, TN: Abingdon Press.

Welch, S.D. (2000). *A Feminist Ethic of Risk*. (Rev. ed.) Minneapolis, MN: Fortress Press.

Williams, B.R. (2004). Dying young, dying poor: A sociological examination of existential suffering among low socioeconomic status patients. *Journal of Palliative Medicine*, 7: 27–37.

Wilson, K.G., D. Curran, and C.J. McPherson. (2005). A burden to others: A common source of distress for the terminally ill. *Cognitive Behavior Therapy*, 34: 115–123.

Wolfe, J., H.E. Grier, N. Klar, S.B. Levin, J.M. Ellenbogen, and S. Salem-Schatz, et al. (2000). Symptoms and suffering at the end of life in children with cancer. *New England Journal of Medicine*, 342: 326–333.

Wolterstorff, N. (1987). *Lament for a Son*. Grand Rapids: Eerdmans. Quoted in S. Hauerwas. *Naming the Silences. God, Medicine, and the Problem of Suffering*, 149–151. London: T & T Clark International, 1990.

Youngner SJ. Who defines futility? Journal of the American Medical Association. 1988; 260: 2094–2095.

Index

Values, cultural, 14
Violence
  failure to relieve pain as, 49
  subjection to, 16
Voice, nursing's, 23
Vulnerability, 49, 61t, 108–109

Weil, Simone, 31
Will of God, 38
Witnessing of suffering, 30–31, 88, 92–93,
    109. *See also* Nurses, suffering of
Women's pain, undertreatment of, 51
Worry, 11t, 61t

RT
84.5
F477
2008

DATE DUE